Richard Mabey, author and broadcaster, writes regularly for The Sunday Times, The Sunday Telegraph and The Independent. He won wide acclaim on the publication of the original Food for Free in 1972, and again with the publication of the full-colour edition in 1989.

His previous books include The Unofficial Countryside, The Common Ground, The Flowering of Britain, The Frampton Flora, Nature Cure and Birds Britannica. In 1986 he was awarded the Whitbread Biography Prize for his biography of Gilbert White. His Flora Britannica, first published in 1996, also won several awards, including the British Book Awards Illustrated Book of the Year, the Botanical Society of the British Isles' President's Award, and was runner-up in the BP Natural World Book of the Year.

Richard is a member of national and local conservation groups, including Common Ground and Plantlife, and lives in Norfolk.

FOOD
for
FREE

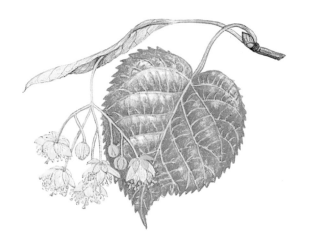

RICHARD MABEY

Collins

For My Mother

HarperCollins Publishers
77-85 Fulham Palace Road
London W6 8JB

The Collins website address is:
www.collins.co.uk

Collins is a registered trademark of HarperCollins Publishers Ltd.

First published in 1972
First full-colour edition published in 1989
This new edition published in 2007

13
10 9 8 7

Text © Richard Mabey 1972, 1989, 2007

Design: Emma Jern and Martin Brown
Editorial Director: Helen Brocklehurst
Editorial: Hugh Brazier, Emily Pitcher and Julia Koppitz
Index: Vanessa Bird

ISBN-13: 978 0 00 724768 4

Collins uses papers that are natural, renewable and recyclable products made from wood grown in sustainable forests. The manufacturing processes conform to the environmental regulations of the country of origin.

Colour reproduction by Colourscan, Singapore
Printed and bound in China by South China Printing Co,. Ltd

Contents

Food for Free is a life-enhancing classic. That it is erudite and charming as well as practical and accurate is a testament to Richard Mabey's great gift as a biographer of our natural heritage. It remains the best possible antidote to the over-processed and the pre-packaged.

Hugh Fearnley-Whittingstall

PREFACE
TO THE NEW EDITION

The first edition of Food for Free was published in 1972 –
a propitious moment, for it coincided with the beginnings of
public concern about both the natural environment and the
quality of our food. Echoes of the sixties were still in the air
– that decade that has become synonymous with youthful
idealism. Reading my text thirty years on I can trace all these
influences, but perhaps the latter most strongly.

I have a snapshot of myself taken around the time the
book was published. I'm sitting cross-legged on the lawn in
a kaftan, and cradling, with something of a smirk on my
face, an immense puffball. Foraging was more than tapping
into some ancient rural heritage. It was cheeky, challenging,
a snub to domesticity as much as domestication. I'd begun
my explorations out of a combination of pure hedonism
and historical curiosity. But I was beginning to feel that
foraging might be a way – at all kinds of social and cultural
and psychological levels – of 'reconnecting with the wild'.

Since then an interest in wild food has, dare one say,
mushroomed. Foraged wildings are now common currency
in TV food programmes and restaurants. Local authorities
lay on guided fungus forays in their country parks. The
seeds of wild vegetables like Good-King-Henry are now
back on the market – in the case of some varieties for the
first time in three centuries. The rise and rise of wild foods
is perfectly expressed by the changing fortunes of that
delectable seashore succulent, marsh samphire. In the sixties
it was an arcane subsistence food, a 'poor man's asparagus'.
In 1981 it was served at Charles and Diana's wedding
breakfast, gathered fresh from the Crown's own marshes at
Sandringham. Now it's a widespread garnish for restaurant

fish, and a favourite seaside holiday souvenir, sold by the bag to those who don't want to get their own legs mud-plastered.

All of which raises still raises, in some minds, the question: Why? Why should twenty-first-century eaters-out, with easy access to most of the taste sensations on the planet, choose to browse about like Palaeolithics? They're opting for the most part for inconvenience food, for bramble-scrabbling, mud-larking, tree-climbing. For the uncomfortable business of peeling horse-radish and de-husking chestnuts. For the sour, the insect-ridden, the misshapen. But of course that is the point. The weather, the landscape, the gratifying discomfort of hunting down your own food the hard way, infuse its whole savour. Henry David Thoreau wrote in Wild Fruits (1859), 'The bitter-sweet of a white-oak acorn which you nibble in a bleak November walk over the tawny earth is more to me than a slice of imported pine-apple.' It's sometimes called the quality of 'gatheredness'.

To judge from the hundreds of letters I've been sent over the years, readers understand this. The intimacy with nature that foraging involves isn't seen as pretend primitivism or some misty-eyed nostalgia for the simple life. Rather, it has encouraged a growing awareness of how food fits into the whole living scheme of things, and a curiosity and inventiveness that are every bit as sharp as our ancestors'. Readers were writing about wild raspberry vinegar long before it became a fashionable ingredient of nouvelle cuisine; about the secret sites and local names of the little wild damsons that grow on the Essex borders; about childhood feasts of seaweed 'boiled in burn water and laid on dog roses to dry'. Foreign cuisines, in which wild plants have always been important ingredients, have been brought to bear on our native wildings, and there have been experiments with fruit liqueurs that go some way beyond sloe gin: service berries in malt whisky, cloudberries in aquavit, gin with extra juniper berries. The whole process of rediscovery has been commemorated in the Suffolk village of Milden, named after that Neolithic staple vegetable fat-hen (melde in Old English), where the parish council has put up a cast-iron statue of their name plant, which the local farmers are forever trying to eradicate from their sugar-beet fields.

Wild foods have now become popular enough to go commercial. There are professional gatherers supplying the restaurant trade. A Scottish brewery uses Argyllshire heather tops to flavour a hugely popular ale sold as leann fraoch. Nettle leaves wrap Cornish harg. Pickled samphire appears on coastal pub counters, alongside the cheese cubes and peanuts. It's wild fungi that have experienced the most dramatic change in image. After centuries of local suspicion, they've been embraced by the supermarkets. One autumn I found twenty-four British species on sale in Harrods.

But it's fungi that raise one of the current worries about foraging. Has it become too popular? In some areas, like the New Forest and Burnham Beeches, commercial mushroom gathering has become so heavy that it has had to be controlled. I've seen wild raspberry bushes trampled into the ground by thoughtless pickers. Even samphire – an annual and therefore dependent on its seed – may be threatened by over-picking along some coastlines. Do we, living in a built-up, over-farmed and over-populated country like Britain, need a kind of foraging ethic, which regulates our leisure whims in keeping with the needs of other organisms in the ecosystem? And, just as foraging is a metaphor for a larger connected relationship with nature, mightn't such an ethic have the rough shape for a model of responsible food consumption?

I've become more of a wayside nibbler than a heavy forager these days. I like serendipitous findings, small wayside gourmet treats. I relish the shock of the new taste, that first bite of the unfamiliar apple. Reed-stems, sucked for their sugary sap. Sun-dried English prunes, from a damson bush strimmed while it was in fruit. Often it is literal apples, wayside wildings sprung from thrown-away cores and bird droppings. They seem to catch everything that's exhilarating about foraging: a sharpness of taste, and of spirit; an echo of the vast, and mostly lost, genetic diversity of cultivated fruits; a sense of place and season. I've found apples that tasted of pears, fizzed like sherbet, smelt of quince. But it's the finding of them, the intimacy with the trees and the places they grow, a heightened consciousness of what they need to survive, that are just as important. And it's maybe that growing sense of intimacy amongst the new foragers that will provide the feedback to conserve their resource: 'If you don't take care of it you lose it.' It could even be a spur to the rewilding of surplus farmland and the revival of responsible common rights. For me, it has generated the rough ethic – or maybe etiquette – of scavenging, or gleaning. For preference I work the margins now, look for windfalls, vegetable road-kills, sudden flushes, leftovers. Or just those small, serendipitous treats off the bush. The 1930s fruit gourmet Edward Bunyan, meandering through his gooseberry patch, described the pleasures of 'ambulant consumption': 'The freedom of the bush should be given to all visitors.' The freedom of the bush – it's a liberty we should all enjoy, but also treasure.

This new edition contains up-to-date nutritional information and many of the ideas sent in by readers. My heartfelt thanks to them and to the HarperCollins editorial team who so skilfully tied them all together. But I have retained the heart of the text, with all its youthful and sometimes naive idealism. That, I feel, is what the book is about. If there are moments of, shall we say, tastelessness as a consequence, then the responsibility is entirely mine.

Richard Mabey, Norfolk, 2006

INTRODUCTION

It is easy to forget, as one stands before the modern supermarket shelf, that every single one of the world's vegetable foods was once a wild plant. What we buy and eat today is still essentially nothing more special than the results of generations of plant-breeding experiments. For most of human history these were directed towards improving size and cropping ability. Some were concerned with flavour and texture – but these are fickle qualities, dependent for their popularity as much on fashion as on any inherent virtue. In later years there have been more ominous moves towards improving colour and shape, and most recently we have seen developments such as genetically modified crop plants and irradiated food, raising worries not only about human health but also about the potentially harmful effects of modern farming methods on the environment.

Indeed, concerns over modern methods of food production have led to something of a backlash, and Michelin-starred chefs are advocating the joys of marsh samphire, a native coastal plant that goes beautifully with another native wild food, fish. For the rest of us likewise: if plant breeding has been directed towards the introduction of bland, inoffensive flavours, and has sacrificed much for the sake of convenience, those old robust tastes, the curly roots and fiddlesome leaves, are still there for the enjoyment of those who care to seek them out.

To some extent, we have become conditioned by the shrink-wrapped, perfectly shaped produce we find in our supermarkets, and we are reluctant to venture into woods, pastures, cliff-tops and marshlands in search of food. But in fact almost every British garden vegetable (greenhouse species excepted) still has a wild ancestor flourishing here. Wild cabbages grow along the south coast, celery along the east. Wild parsnips flourish on waste ground everywhere. Historically these have always been sources of food in times of scarcity, yet each time with less ingenuity and confidence, less native knowledge about what they are and how they can be used.

Food for Free is about these plants, and how they once were and can still be used as food. It is a practical book, I hope, though it would be foolish to pretend that there are any pressing economic reasons why we should have a large-scale revival of wild food use. You would need to be a most determined picker to keep yourself alive on wild vegetables, and since they are so easy to cultivate there would be very little point in trying. Nor are wild fruits and vegetables necessarily more healthy and nutritious than cultivated varieties – though some are, and most of them are likely to be comparatively free of herbicides and other agricultural poisons.

Why bother, then? Why not leave wild food utterly to the birds and slugs? My initial pleas are, I'm afraid, almost purely sensual and indulgent: interest, experience, and even, on a small scale, adventure. The history of wild food use is interesting enough in its own right, and those who would never dream of grubbing about on a damp woodland floor for their supper may still find themselves impressed by our ancestors' resourcefulness. But those who are prepared to venture out will find more substantial rewards. It is the flavours and textures that will surprise the most, I think, and the realisation of to just what extent the cultivation and mass production of food have muted our taste experiences. There is a whole galaxy of powerful and surprising flavours preserved intact in the wild stock that are quite untapped in cultivated foods: tart and smoky berries, aromatic fungi, crisp and succulent shoreline plants.

There is much along these lines that could be said in favour of wild foods. Some of them are delicacies, many of them are still abundant, and all of them are free. They require none of the attention demanded by garden plants, and possess the additional attraction of having to be found. I think I would rate this as perhaps the most attractive single feature of wild food use. The satisfactions of cultivation are slow and measured. They are not at all like the excitement of raking through a rich bed of cockles, of suddenly discovering a clump of sweet cicely, of tracking down a bog myrtle by its smell alone. There is something akin to hunting here: the search, the gradually acquired wisdom about seasons and habitats, the satisfaction of having proved you can provide for yourself. What you find may make no more than an intriguing addition to your normal diet, but it was you that found it. And in coastal areas, in a good autumn, it could be a whole three-course meal.

Wild food and necessity

It is not easy to tell how wide a range of plants was eaten before agriculture began. The seeds of any number of species have been found in Neolithic settlements, but these may have already been under a primitive system of cultivation. Plants gathered from the wild would inevitably drop their seed and begin to grow near their pickers' dwellings; and if, as was likely, the specimens collected were above average in size or yield, so might be their offspring. So a sort of automatic selection would have taken place, with crops of the more fruitful plants growing naturally near habitation.

By the Elizabethan era, the range of wild plants and herbs used and understood by the average cottager was wide and impressive. In many ways it had to be. There was no other source of readily available medicine, or of many fruits and vegetables. Yet even under conditions of necessity, how is one to explain the discovery that as cryptic a part as the styles of the saffron crocus was useful as a spice? The number of wild bits and pieces that must have been put to the test in the kitchen at one time or another is hair-raising. We should be thankful the job has been done for us.

Many plants passed into use as food at this time as a by-product of their medicinal use. Black currants, for instance, were certainly used for throat lotions before the recipients realised they were also quite pleasant to eat when you were well. Sheer economy also played a part, as in finding a use for hop tops that had to be thinned out in the spring.

But like so much else, these old skills and customs were eroded by industrialisation and the drift to the towns. The process was especially thorough in the case of wild foods because cultivation brought genuine advances in quality and abundance. But if the knowledge of how to use them was fading, the plants themselves continued to thrive. Most of them prospered as they had always done in woods and hedgerows. Those that flourished best in the human habitats bided their time under fields which had been turned over to cultivation, or moved into the new wasteland habitats that were a by-product of urbanisation. Plants which had been introduced as pot-herbs clung on at the edges of gardens, as persistent as weeds as they were once abundant as vegetables.

Then some crisis would strike the conventional food supplies, and people would be thankful for this persistence. On the island fringes of Britain, where the ground is poor and the weather unpredictably hostile, the tough native plants were the only invariably successful crops. The knowledge of how to use these plants as emergency rations was kept right up to the time air transport provided a reliable lifeline to the mainland.

It was the two World Wars, and the disruptions of food supplies that accompanied them, which provided one of the most striking examples of the usefulness of wild foods. All over occupied Europe fungi were gathered from woods, and wild greens from bomb sites. In America, pilots were given instructions on how to live off the wild in case their planes were ditched over land. And in this country, the government encouraged the 'hedgerow harvest' (as they called one of their publications) as much as the growing of carrots.

Wild plants are invaluable during times of famine or crisis, precisely because they are wild. They are quickly available, tough, resilient, resistant to disease, adapted to the climate and soil conditions. If they were not, they would have simply failed to survive. They are always there, waiting for their moment, thriving under conditions that our pampered cultivated plants would find intolerable.

Some modern agriculturalists are beginning to look seriously at these special qualities of wild food plants. Conventional agriculture works by taking an end food product as given, and modifying plants and conditions of growth to produce it as efficiently as possible. In regions that are vastly different from the plant's natural environment, its survival is always precarious, and often at damaging expense to the soil and the natural environment. The alternative approach is to study the plants that grow naturally and luxuriantly in the area, and see what possible food products can be obtained from them. This should become an especially fruitful line of research in developing countries with poor soils.

Plant use and conservation

These last few instances are examples of conditions in which wild food use was anything but a frivolous pastime.

I sincerely hope that this book will never be needed as a manual for that sort of situation. But is there really nothing more to gathering wild foods than the fun of the hunt, and the promise of some exotic new flavours? I think there is. Getting to know these plants and the uses that have been made of them is to begin to understand a whole section of our social history. The plants are a museum in themselves, hangovers from times when palates were less fastidious, living records of famines and changing fashions and even whole peoples. To know their history is to understand how intricately food is bound up with the whole pattern of our social lives. It is easy to forget this by the supermarket shelf, where the food is instantly and effortlessly available, and soil and labour seem part of another existence. We take our food for granted as we do our air and water, and all three are threatened as a result.

Yet familiarity with the ways of just a few of the plants in this book gives an insight at first hand into the complex and delicate relationships which plants have with their environment: their dependence on birds to carry their seeds, on animals to crop the grass that shuts out their light, on wind and sunshine and the balance of chemicals in the soil, and ultimately on our own good grace as to whether they survive at all. It is on the products, wild or cultivated, of this intricate network of forces that our food resources depend.

I know there may be some people who will object to this book on the grounds that it may encourage further depletions of our dwindling wildlife. I believe that the exact opposite is true. One of the major problems in conservation today is not how to keep people insulated from nature but how to help them engage more closely with it, so that they can appreciate its value and vulnerability, and the way its needs can be reconciled with those of humans. One of the most complex and intimate relationships which most of us can have with the natural environment is to eat it. I hope I am not overstating my case when I say that to follow this relationship through personally, from the search to the cooking pot, is a more practical lesson than most in the economics of the natural world. Far from encouraging rural vandalism, it helps deepen respect for the interdependence of all living things. At the very least it will provide a strong motive for looking after particular species and maybe individual ecosystems.

And maybe foraging can contribute even more, in today's ecologically threatened world. If plants like wilding apples could contribute to the restoration of lost cultivated varieties, maybe, conversely, the restoration of cultivated land to wild, forageable land could build up new natural ecosystems. The possibility of the revival of a gentle communal use of such places would add foraging to the increasing range of community food initiatives, from organic food boxes to city farms.

Omissions

This book covers the majority of wild plant food products which can be obtained in the British Isles. But there are some categories which I have deliberately omitted.

- There is nothing on grasses and cereals. This is intended to be a practical book, and no one is going to spend their time hand-gathering enough wild seeds to make flour.
- I have touched briefly on the traditional herbal uses of many plants where this is relevant or interesting. But I have included no plants purely on the grounds of their presumed therapeutic value. This is a book about food, not medicine.
- This is also a book about wild plant foods, which is the simple reason (apart from personal qualms) why there is nothing about fish and wildfowl.

- But I have included shellfish because, from a picker's perspective, they are more like plants than animals. They stay more or less in one place, and are gathered, not caught.

Layout of the book

The text is divided into sections covering (1) edible plants (trees and herbaceous plants, including one fern), (2) fungi and lichens, (3) seaweeds, (4) shellfish. Within each category, species are arranged in systematic order.

SOME PICKING RULES

I have given more detailed notes on gathering techniques in the introductions to the individual sections (particularly fungi, seaweeds and shellfish). But there are some general rules which apply to all wild food. Following these rules will help to guarantee the quality of what you are picking, and the health of the plant, fungus or shellfish population that is providing it.

Although we have tried to make both text and illustrations as helpful as possible in identifying the different plant products described in this book, they should not be regarded as a substitute for a comprehensive field guide. They will help you decide what to gather, but until you are experienced it is wise to double-check everything (particularly fungi) in a book devoted solely to identification. Conversely, never rely on illustrations alone as a guide to edibility. Some of the plants illustrated here need the special preparation described in the text before they are palatable.

But although it is obviously crucial to know what you are picking, don't become obsessed about the possible dangers of poisoning. This is a natural worry when you are trying wild foods for the first time, but happily a groundless one. As you will see from the text there are relatively few common poisonous plants and fungi in Britain compared with the total number of plant species.

To put the dangers of wild foods into perspective it is worth considering the trials attendant on eating the cultivated foods we stuff into our mouths without question. Forgetting for a moment the perennial problems of additives and insecticide residues, and the new worries about irradiated and genetically modified food, how many people know that, in excess, cabbage can cause goitre and onions induce anaemia? That as little as one whole nutmeg can bring on days of hallucinations? Almost any food substance can occasionally bring on an allergic reaction in a susceptible subject, and oysters and strawberries, as well as nuts of all types, have particularly infamous reputations in this respect. But all these effects are rare. The point is that they are part of the hazards of eating itself, rather than of a particular category of food.

Here are some basic rules to ensure your safety when gathering and using wild foods:
- Make sure you correctly identify the plant, fungus or seaweed you are gathering.
- Do not gather any sort of produce from areas that may have been sprayed with insecticide or weedkiller.
- Avoid, too, the verges of heavily used roads, where the plant may have been contaminated by car exhausts. There are plenty of environments that are likely to be comparatively free of all types of contamination: commons, woods, the hedges along footpaths, etc. Even in a small garden you are likely to be able to find

something like twenty of the species described in this book.

- Wherever possible use a flat open basket to gather your produce, to avoid squashing. If you are caught without a basket, and do not mind being folksy, pin together some dock or burdock leaves with thorns.
- When you have got the crop home, wash it well and sort out any old or decayed parts.
- To be doubly sure, it is as well to try fairly small portions of new foods the first time you eat them, just to ensure that you are not sensitive to them.

Having considered your own survival, consider the plant's:

- Never strip a plant of leaves, berries, or whatever part you are picking. Take small quantities from each specimen, so that its appearance and health are not affected. It helps to use a knife or scissors (except with fungi: see p. 184).
- Never take the flowers or seeds of annual plants; they rely on them for survival.
- Do not take more than you need for your own needs.
- Never pull up whole plants along any path or road verge where the public has access. It is not only antisocial and contrary to all the principles of conservation, but also, in most places, illegal.
- Under the Wildlife and Countryside Act it is illegal to dig up a plant by the root, however common it is, unless it is on your own land or you have the landowner's permission.
- Be careful not to damage other vegetation or surrounding habitat when gathering wild food.
- Adhere at all times to the Code of Conduct for the conservation and enjoyment of wild plants, published by the Botanical Society of the British Isles (**www.bsbi.org.uk/Code.htm**).

CALENDAR

A month-by-month guide to the availability of some of the
wild foods mentioned in this book.

January
Chickweed
Oyster mushroom
Velvet shank

February
Chickweed
Garlic mustard
Stinging nettle
Velvet shank

March
Common comfrey
Garlic mustard
Hop shoots
Morel
Stinging nettle
Sweet violet
Velvet shank

April
Bistort
Carrageen
Cow parsley
Dandelion flowers
Fairy-ring champignon
Hawthorn leaves
Hop shoots
Morel
Stinging nettle
Ramsons
Sea beet
St George's mushroom
Sweet violet
Tansy leaves

May
Carrageen
Dandelion flowers
Fairy-ring
  champignon
Hop shoots
Morel
Stinging nettle
Ramsons
Sea beet
St George's mushroom
Sweet violet
Woodruff

June

Elderflowers
Fairy-ring champignon
Marsh samphire
Ramsons
Stinging nettle
Sea beet
Shaggy inkcap
St George's mushroom
Wild rose flowers
Wild strawberry
Wild thyme

July

Black currant
Chanterelle
Fairy-ring champignon
Field mushroom
Giant puffball
Gooseberry
Horse mushroom
Lime blossom
Marsh samphire
Parasol mushroom
Raspberry
Red currant
Sea beet
Shaggy inkcap
Walnut, green
Wild marjoram
Wild rose flowers
Wild strawberry
Wild thyme

August

Bilberry
Black mustard seeds
Blackberry
Cauliflower fungus
Cep
Chanterelle
Elderberries
Fairy-ring champignon
Field mushroom
Giant puffball
Gooseberry
Hazelnut
Heather flowers
Horse mushroom
Parasol mushroom
Raspberry
Rosehip
Sea beet
Shaggy inkcap
Wild marjoram
Wild strawberry
Wild thyme
Wood hedgehog

September

Beech nuts
Beefsteak fungus
Bilberry
Black mustard seeds
Blackberry
Blewit
Cauliflower fungus

Cep
Chanterelle
Common poppy seeds
Dandelion roots
Elderberries
Fairy-ring champignon
Field mushroom
Garlic mustard
Giant puffball
Hawthorn berries
Hazelnut
Heather flowers
Honey fungus
Hop fruits
Horse mushroom
Juniper
Parasol mushroom
Raspberry
Rosehip
Rowan
Saffron milk cap
Sea beet
Shaggy inkcap
Velvet shank
Wild service-tree
Wild strawberry
Wood hedgehog

Cauliflower fungus
Cep
Chanterelle
Chickweed
Elderberries
Fairy-ring champignon
Field mushroom
Garlic mustard
Giant puffball
Hazelnut
Honey fungus
Horse mushroom
Jew's ear
Juniper
Oyster mushroom
Parasol mushroom
Rosehip
Rowan
Saffron milk cap
Sea beet
Shaggy inkcap
Sloe
Sweet chestnut
Velvet shank
Walnut, ripe
Wood hedgehog

October

Beech nuts
Beefsteak fungus
Blackberry
Blewit

November

Blewit
Cauliflower fungus
Cep
Chanterelle
Chickweed

Fairy-ring champignon
Field mushroom
Giant puffball
Honey fungus
Horse mushroom
Jew's ear
Medlar (after first frost)
Oyster mushroom
Rosehip
Saffron milk cap
Shaggy inkcap
Sweet chestnut
Velvet shank
Walnut, ripe
Wood hedgehog

December

Blewit
Chanterelle
Chickweed
Fairy-ring champignon
Honey fungus
Oyster mushroom
Velvet shank

Edible plants

Roots

Roots are probably the least practical of all wild vegetables. Firstly, few species form thick, fleshy roots in the wild, and the coarse, wiry roots of – for instance – horse-radish and wild parsnip are really only suitable for flavouring. Second, under the Wildlife and Countryside Act it is illegal to dig up wild plants by the root, except on your own land, or with the permission of the landowner.

The few species that are subsequently recommended as roots are all very common and likely to crop up as garden weeds. Where palatable roots of a practical size and texture can be found, however, they are quite versatile, and may be used in the preparation of broths (herb-bennet), vegetable dishes (large-flowered evening-primrose), salads (oxeye daisy), or even drinks (chicory, dandelion).

Green vegetables

The main problem with wild leaf vegetables is their size. Not many wild plants have the big, floppy leaves for which cultivated greens have been bred, and as a result picking enough for a serving can be a long and irksome task. For this reason the optimum picking time for most leaf vegetables is probably their middle-age, when the flowers are out and the plant is easy to recognise, and the leaves have reached maximum size without beginning to wither.

Green vegetables can be roughly divided into three types: salads, cooked greens, and stems. For general recipes see dandelion (p. 169) for salads, sea beet (p. 71) or fat-hen (p. 67) for greens, and alexanders (p. 133) for stems.

All green vegetables can also be made into soup (see sorrel, p. 79), blended into green sauces, or made into a pottage or 'mess of greens' by cooking a number of species together.

Herbs

A herb is generally defined as a leafy plant used not as a food in its own right but as a flavouring for other foods, and most herbs tend to be milder in the wild state than under domestication; being valued principally for their flavouring qualities, it is these which domestication has attempted to intensify, not delicacy, size, succulence or any of the other qualities that are sought after in staple vegetables. You will find, consequently, that with wild herbs you will need to double up the quantities you normally use of the cultivated variety.

The best time to pick a herb, especially for the purposes of drying, is just as it is coming into flower. This is the stage at which the plant's nutrients and aromatic oils are still mainly concentrated in the leaves, yet it will have a few blossoms to assist with the identification. Gather your herbs in dry weather and preferably early in the morning before they have been exposed to too much sun. Wet herbs will tend to develop mildew during drying, and specimens picked after long exposure to strong sunshine will inevitably have lost some of their natural oils by evaporation.

Cut whole stalks of the herb with a knife or scissors to avoid damaging the parent plant. If you are going to use the herbs fresh, strip the leaves and flowers off the stalks as soon as you get them home. If you are going to dry them, leave the stalks intact as you have picked them. To maintain their colour and flavour they must be dried as quickly as possible but without too intense a heat. They therefore need a combination of gentle warmth and good ventilation. A kitchen or well-ventilated airing cupboard is ideal. The stalks can be hung up in loose bunches, or spread thinly on a sheet of paper and placed on the rack above the stove. Ideally, they should also be covered by muslin, to keep out flies and insects and, in the case of hanging bundles, to catch any leaves that start to crumble and fall as they dry. All herbs can be used to flavour vinegar, olive oil or drinks, as with thyme in aquavit.

Spices

Spices are the aromatic seeds of flowering plants. There are also a few roots (most notably horse-radish) that are generally regarded as spices.

Most plants which have aromatic leaves also have aromatic seeds, and can be usefully employed as flavourings. But a warning: do not expect the flavour of the two parts to be identical. They are often subtly different in ways that make it inadvisable simply to substitute seeds for leaves.

Seeds should always be allowed to dry on the plant. After flowering, annuals start to concentrate their food supplies into the seeds so that they have enough to survive through germination. This also, of course, increases the flavour and size of the seeds. When they are dry and ready to drop off the plant, their food content and flavour should be at a maximum.

Flowers

Gathering wild flowers for no other reason than their diverting flavours would at least be antisocial, and in the case of the rarest species it is illegal under the Wildlife and

Countryside Act. Some of the flowers mentioned in this book are rare and should not be picked these days because of declining populations, though many of them have been anciently popular ingredients of salads, and are included for their historical interest.

The only species I advocate picking from are those where removing flowers in small quantities is unlikely to have much visual or biological effect. They are all common and hardy plants. They are all perennials and do not rely on seeding for continued survival. They are mostly bushes or shrubs in which each individual produces an abundant number of blossoms.

Most of the recipes in the book require no more than a handful or two of blossoms, but if you like the sound of any of them it may be best to grow the plants in your garden and pick the flowers there. Many species, such as cowslip and primrose, are commercially available as seed.

Fruits

A number of the fruits I have included are cultivated and used commercially as well as growing in the wild. Where this is the case I have not given much space to the more common kitchen uses, which can be found in any cookery book. I have concentrated instead on how to find and gather the wild varieties, and on the more unusual traditional recipes.

Almost all fruit, of course, can be used to make jellies and jams. Rather than repeat the relevant directions under each fruit, it is useful to go into some detail here. The notes below apply to all species.

Another process which can be applied to most of the harder-skinned fruits is drying. Choose slightly unripe fruit, wash well, and dry with a cloth. Then strew it out on a metal tray and place in a very low oven (50 °C, 120 °F). The fruit is dry when it yields no juice when squeezed between the fingers, but is not so far gone that it rattles. This usually takes between 4 and 6 hours.

Most of the fruits in this section can also be used to make wine (not covered in this book); fruit liqueurs (see, for example, sloe gin, p. 47); flavoured vinegars (see raspberry, p. 109); pies, fools (see gooseberry, p. 106); summer or autumn puddings (see raspberry, p. 109, and blackberry, p. 111).

Some fruits, notable the medlar and the fruit of the service-tree, need to be 'bletted' – in other words, half-rotten – before they are edible.

Making a jelly

Jellies and jams form because of a chemical reaction between a substance called pectin, present in the fruit, and sugar. The pectin (and the fruit's acids, which also play a part in the reaction) tend to be most concentrated when the fruit is under-ripe. But then of course the flavour is only partly developed. So the optimum time for picking fruit for jelly is when it is just ripe.

The amount of pectin available varies from fruit to fruit. Apples, gooseberries and currants, for instance, are rich in pectin and acid and set very readily. Blackberries and strawberries, on the other hand, have a low pectin content, and usually need to have some added from an outside source before they will form a jelly. Lemon juice or sour crab apples are commonly used for this.

The first stage in making a jelly is to pulp the fruit. Do this by packing the clean fruit into a saucepan or preserving pan and just covering with water. Bring to the boil and simmer until all the fruit is mushy. With the harder-skinned fruits (rosehips, haws, etc.) you may need to help the process along by pressing with a spoon, and be prepared to simmer for up to half an hour. This is the stage to supplement the pectin, if your fruit has poor setting properties. Add the juice of one lemon for every 900 g (2 lb) of fruit.

When you have your pulp, separate the juice from the roughage and fibres by straining through muslin. This can be done by lining a large bowl with a good-sized sheet of muslin, folded at least double, and filling the bowl with the fruit pulp. Then lift and tie the corners of the muslin, using the back of a chair or a low clothes line as the support, so that it hangs like a sock above the bowl. Alternatively, use a real stocking, or a purpose-made straining bag.

To obtain the maximum volume of juice, allow the pulp to strain overnight. It is not too serious to squeeze the muslin if you are in a hurry, but it will force some of the solid matter through and affect the clarity of the jelly. When you have all the juice you want, measure its volume, and transfer it to a clean saucepan, adding 500 g (1 lb) of sugar for every 500 ml (1 pint) of juice. Bring to the boil, stirring well, and boil rapidly, skimming off any scum that floats to the surface. A jelly will normally form when the mixture has reached a temperature of 105 °C (221 °F) on a jam thermometer. If you have no thermometer, or want a confirmatory test, transfer one drop of the mixture with a spoon onto a cold saucer. If setting is imminent, the drop will not run after a few seconds because of a skin – often visible – formed across it.

As soon as the setting temperature has been achieved, pour the mixture into some clear, warm jars (preferably standing on a metal surface to conduct away some of the heat). Cover the surface of the jelly with a wax disc, wax side down. Add a cellophane cover, moistening it on the outside first so that it dries taut. Hold the cover in place with a rubber band, label the jar clearly, and store in a cool place.

Nuts

The majority of plants covered by this book are in the 'fruit and veg' category. They make perfectly acceptable accompaniments or conclusions to a meal, but would leave you feeling a little peckish if you relied on nothing else. Nuts are an exception. They are the major source of second-class protein amongst wild plants. Walnuts, for instance, contain 18 per cent protein, 60 per cent fat, and can provide over 600 kilocalories per 100 grams of kernels.

It is therefore possible to substitute nuts for the more conventional protein constituents of a meal, as indeed vegetarians have been doing for centuries. But do not pick them to excess because of this. Wild nuts are crucial to the survival of many wild birds and animals, who have just as much right to them, and considerably more need.

Keep those you do pick very dry, for damp and mould can easily permeate nutshells and rot the kernel.

As well as being edible in their natural state, nuts may be eaten pickled or puréed, mixed into salads, or as a main constituent of vegetable dishes.

TREES

• •

Juniper
Juniperus communis

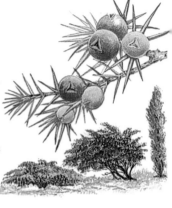

Locally common on chalk downs, limestone hills, heaths and moors, chiefly in southeast England and the north. A shrub 1.5–3.5 m (4–12 ft) high – though there is also a prostrate form – with whorls of narrow evergreen leaves. Flowers, small, yellow, at the base of the leaves, appear in May and June. The fruit is a green berry-like cone, appearing in June but not ripening until September or October of its second year, when it turns blue-black.

At the time of ripening, juniper berries are rich in oil, which is the source of their use as a flavouring. They are of course best known as the flavouring in gin, and most of the historical uses have been in one kind of drink or another (though home-grown berries have not been used by British distillers for over a century). Experiment with drinks in which the berries have been steeped. Even gin is improved by, as it were, a double dose.

Uses across Europe are varied. They have been roasted and ground as a coffee substitute. In Sweden they are used to make a type of beer, and are often turned into jam. In France, *genevrette* is made by fermenting a mixture of juniper berries and barley.

Crushed juniper berries are becoming increasingly popular as a flavouring for white meat or game dishes. In Belgium they are used to make a sauce for pork chops. Seal the chops on both sides and place in a shallow casserole. Sprinkle with lemon juice and add parsley, four crushed juniper berries, rosemary, salt and pepper. Arrange peeled and sliced apples over the top and then pour over melted butter. Cook in a medium oven for 30 minutes.

Hop
Humulus lupulus

A familiar perennial climber, 3–6 m (10–20 ft) high. Locally frequent in hedges, woodland edges and damp thickets, especially in the southern half of England. Flowers July to August.

The green, cone-like female flowers of the hop have been used in mainland Europe for flavouring beer since the ninth century. Although the plant is a British native, hops were not used for brewing in this country until the fifteenth century. Even then there was considerable opposition to their addition to the old ale recipes, and it was another hundred years before hop-growing became a commercial operation.

Wild hops can be used for home brewing, but a more intriguing and possibly older custom makes use of the very young shoots and leaves, picked not later than May. They may be an ancient wild vegetable, but most of the recipes came into being as a way of making frugal use of the mass of trimmings produced when the hop plantations were pruned in the spring.

The shoots can be chopped up and simmered in butter as a sauce, added to soups and omelettes, or, most popularly, cooked like asparagus. For the latter, strip the young shoots of the larger leaves, tie them in bundles and soak in salt water for an hour, drain and then plunge into boiling water for a few minutes until just tender. Serve with molten butter.

Hop frittata

Frittata is an Italian recipe that can be used with many of the green-stem wild vegetables in this book – for example, asparagus, wild garlic, thistles and bramble shoots. A frittata should be much more solid than an omelette, and can be served hot or cold.

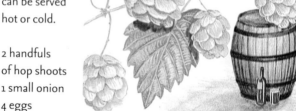

2 handfuls
of hop shoots
1 small onion
4 eggs
1 dessertspoon dried breadcrumbs
1 dessertspoon parmesan cheese
Parsley

1 Beat the eggs with seasoning to taste, and with the breadcrumbs and parmesan cheese.
2 Chop the hop shoots into roughly 5 cm (2 inch) lengths and fry with the chopped onion in a little olive oil in a heavy pan until they have both begun to brown.
3 Add the beaten egg mixture and simmer over a low heat. In about four or five minutes the frittata should have set.
4 Take a large plate, cover the pan and turn over so that the frittata settles onto it. Then slide it back into the pan, and simmer until the other side is brown.

Walnut

Juglans regia

Deciduous tree, up to 30 m (100 ft) high, with grey, fissured bark. Leaves are odd-pinnate, with 5 to 9 leaflets. Catkins followed by flowers. Nuts ripen in September.

The walnut is a native of southern Europe, introduced to this country some 500 years ago for its wood and its fruit. Although not quick to spread outside cultivation, there are some self-sown trees in warm spots such as hedgerows, and seeds can be carried away from the parent trees by birds and mammals.

Walnuts are best when they are fairly ripe and dry, in late October and November. Before this, the young 'wet' walnuts are rather tasteless. If you wish to pick them young, do so in July whilst they are still green and make pickle from them. They should be soft enough to pass a skewer through. Prick them lightly with a fork to allow the pickle to permeate the skin, and leave them to stand in strong brine for about a week, until they are quite black. Drain and wash them and let them dry for two or three days more. Pack them into jars and cover them with hot pickling vinegar. Seal the jars and allow to stand for at least a month before eating.

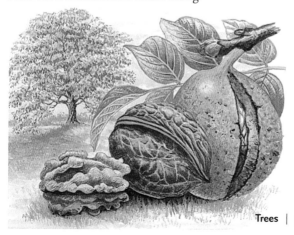

Mushroom cutlets with walnut cream sauce

Chop the mushrooms finely, cook in a little butter and drain. Soak 125 g (5 oz) of soft breadcrumbs in milk and squeeze dry. Dice and sauté an onion, beat together two eggs and chop some parsley. Combine all the ingredients, form into cutlets and fry in oil. Finally, chop the walnuts with a little more parsley, blend with cream and season.

• •

Beech
Fagus sylvatica

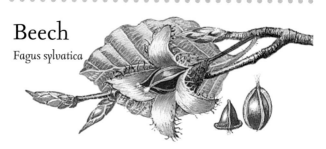

Widespread and common throughout the British Isles, especially on chalky soils. A stately tree, up to 40 m (130 ft), with smooth grey bark and leaves of a bright, translucent green. Nuts in September and October, four inside a prickly brown husk. When ripe this opens into four lobes, thus liberating the brown, three-sided nuts.

Beech dominates the chalk soils of southern England and is associated with a number of species of fungi. It is a native species, and has long provided a source of fuel, although it did not gain popularity as a material for furniture until the eighteenth century. Since then it has become extremely popular in the kitchen – albeit for building kitchen units rather than for its culinary delights.

However, the botanical name *Fagus* originates from a Greek word meaning to eat, though in the case of the beech this is likely to have referred to pigs rather than to humans.

This is not to say that beechmast – the usual term for the nuts – is disagreeable. Raw, or roasted and salted, it tastes not unlike young walnut. But the nuts are very small, and the collection and peeling of enough to make an acceptable meal is a tiresome business.

This is also an obstacle to the rather more interesting use of beechmast as a source of vegetable oil. Although I have never tried the extraction process myself, mainly because of a lack of suitable equipment, it has been widely used in mainland Europe, particularly in times of economic hardship, such as in Germany between the two World Wars. Although beech trees generally only fruit every three or four years, each tree produces a prodigious quantity of mast, and there is rarely any difficulty in finding enough. It should be gathered as early as possible, before the squirrels have taken it, and before it has had a chance to dry out. The three-faced nuts should be cleaned of any remaining husks, dirt or leaves and then ground, shells and all, in a small oil-mill. (For those with patience, a mincing machine or a strong blender should work as well.) The resulting pulp should be put inside a fine muslin bag and then in a press or under a heavy weight to extract the oil.

For those able to get this far, the results should be worthwhile. Every 500 g (1 lb) of nuts yields as much as 85 ml (3 fl oz) of oil. The oil itself is rich in fats and proteins, and provided it is stored in well-sealed containers it will keep fresh considerably longer than many other vegetable fats.

Beechnut oil can be used for salads or for frying, like any other cooking oil. Its most exotic application is probably beechnut butter, which is still made in some rural districts in the USA, and for which there was a patent issued in this country during the reign of George I.

In April the young leaves of the beech tree are almost translucent. They shine in the sun from the light passing through them. To touch they are silky, and tear like delicately thin rubber. It is difficult not to want to chew a few as you walk through a beech-wood in spring. And, fresh from the tree, they are indeed a fine salad vegetable, as sweet as a mild cabbage though much softer in texture.

Beech-leaf noyau

An unusual way of utilising beech leaves is to make a potent liqueur called beech-leaf noyau. This probably originated in the Chilterns, where large plantations of beech were put down in the eighteenth and nineteenth centuries to service the chair-making trade. Pack an earthenware or glass jar about nine-tenths full of young, clean leaves. Pour gin into the jar, pressing the leaves down all the time, until they are just covered. Leave to steep for about a fortnight. Then strain off the gin, which will by now have caught the brilliant green of the leaves. To every 500 ml (1 pint) of gin add about 300 g (12 oz) of sugar (more if you like your liqueurs very syrupy) dissolved in 250 ml (1/2 pint) of boiling water, and a dash of brandy. Mix the warm syrup with the gin and bottle as soon as cold. The result is a thickish, sweet spirit, mild and slightly oily to taste, like sake.

• •

Sweet Chestnut

Castanea sativa

Well distributed throughout England, though scattered in Scotland. Common in woods and parks. A tall, straight tree, up to 30 m (100 ft), with single spear-shaped serrated leaves. Nuts in October and November, two or three carried in spherical green cases covered with long spines.

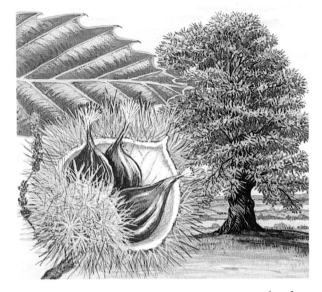

A nut to get your teeth into. And a harvest to get your hands into, if the year is good and the nuts thick enough on the ground to warrant a small sack rather than a basket. Although the tree was in all probability introduced to this country by the Romans, nothing seems more English than gathering and roasting chestnuts on fine autumn afternoons.

The best chestnut trees are the straight, old ones whose leaves turn brown early. Do not confuse them with horse-chestnuts (Aesculus hippocastanum), whose inedible conkers look rather similar to sweet chestnuts inside their spiny husks. In fact the trees are not related, Castanea sativa being more closely related to the oak. They will be covered with the prickly fruit as early as September, and small specimens of the nuts to come will be blown down early in the next month. Ignore them, unless you can find some bright green ones which have just fallen. They are undeveloped and will shrivel within a day or two.

The ripe nuts begin to fall late in October, and can be helped on their way with a few judiciously thrown sticks. Opening the prickly husks can be a painful business, and for the early part of the crop it is as well to take a pair of gloves and some strong boots, the latter for splitting the husks underfoot, the former for extricating the fruits. The polished brown surface of the ripe nuts uncovered by the split husk is positively alluring. You will want to stamp on every husk you see, and rummage down through the leaves and spines to see if the reward is glinting there.

Don't shy away from eating the nuts raw. If the stringy pith is peeled away as well as the shell, most of their bitterness will go. But roasting transforms them. They take on the sweetness and bulk of some tropical fruit. As is the case with so much else in this book, the excitement lies as much in the rituals of preparation as in the food itself. Chestnut roasting is an institution, rich with associations of smell, and of welcomingly hot coals in cold streets. To do it efficiently at home, slit the skins, and put the nuts in the hot ash of an open fire or close to the red coals – save one, which is put in uncut. When this explodes, the others are ready. The explosion is fairly ferocious, scattering hot shrapnel over the room, so sit well back from the fire and make sure all the other nuts have been slit.

Chestnuts are highly versatile. They can be pickled, candied, or made into an amber with breadcrumbs and egg yolk. Boiled with Brussels sprouts they were Goethe's favourite dish. Chopped, stewed and baked with red cabbage, they make a rich vegetable pudding.

Chestnut purée
Chestnut purée is a convenient form in which to use the nuts. Shell and peel the chestnuts. This is easily done if you boil them for 5 minutes first. Boil the shelled nuts again in a thin stock for about 40 minutes. Strain off the liquid and then rub the nuts through a sieve, or mash them in a liquidiser. The resulting purée can be seasoned and used as a substitute for potatoes, or it can form the basis of stuffings, soups and sweets, such as chestnut fool.

Chestnut flour

A more elaborate way of storing the raw material of the nuts is to turn them into flour, as is done in many areas around the Mediterranean. You will need to collect a good number of young chestnuts and store them in a warm, dry and well-ventilated room for a couple of months. Then they must be individually shelled, roasted and ground as finely as possible (a blender is the best way). The resulting yellowish flour is slightly fragrant and excellent in cakes and breads. But it can be reluctant to rise, and is probably best mixed half-and-half with ordinary wheat flour.

Oak

Quercus robur / Quercus petraea

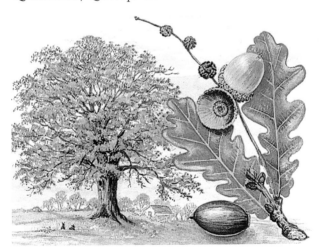

A common deciduous tree up to 35 m (115 ft) high, typically with a broad, domed crown. The two common species are pedunculate oak (Quercus robur), which occurs throughout Britain, and sessile oak

(Q. petraea), which is the dominant species in northern and western Britain, and in Ireland. Leaves are distinctively shaped, with irregular lobes. The fruits (acorns) ripen in September to October.

The oak tree has formed part of our folklore and history for centuries, not only as a source of timber for building houses and ships but also as a source of food. Like beechmast, however, the chief economic use of acorns has been as animal fodder, and they have been used as human food chiefly in times of famine. The raw kernels are forbiddingly bitter to most palates, but chopped and roasted they can be used as a substitute for almonds.

In Europe the most common use of acorns has been to roast them as a substitute for coffee, and they were recommended for this role during the Second World War. Chop the kernels, roast to a light brown colour, grind up, then roast again.

Hazel
Corylus avellana

An abundant and widespread tree, found in woods, hedgerows and scrubland. A small tree or multi-stemmed shrub, 1.5–3.5 m (4–12 ft) high, with roundish, downy, toothed leaves. Well known for the yellow male catkins, called 'lambs' tails', which appear in the winter. Nuts from late August to October, 1–2.5 cm (^{1}/$_2$–1 inch) long, ovoid and encased in a thick green lobed husk.

The hazel was among the first species to recolonise the British Isles after the last Ice Age. It is an extremely useful tree, with leaves that can be used as food for livestock, branches for building fences and shelters, and nuts that can be eaten as food. Widely eaten in prehistoric times, the hazelnut even became part of Celtic legend – its compact shape, hard shell and nutritious fruit was an emblem of concentrated wisdom. Today they are grown commercially in many parts of the world, and are second only to the almond as a world nut crop.

Hazelnuts begin to ripen in mid-September, at about the same time that the leaves begin to yellow. You may have to compete with the birds and squirrels, as the nuts do not just provide a treat for humans. Look for them at the edges of woods and in mature hedges. Search inside bushes for the nuts, as well as working round them, and scan them with the sun behind you if possible. Use a walking stick to bend down the branches, and gather the nuts into a basket that stays open whilst you are picking: a plastic bag with one handle looped over your picking wrist is a useful device.

If the ground cover under the bush is relatively clear or grass, then it is worthwhile giving the bush a shake. Some of the invisible ripe nuts should find their way onto the ground after this. In fact it is always worth searching the ground underneath a hazel. If there are nuts there which are dark or grey-brown in colour then the kernels will have turned to dust. But there is a chance that there will also be fresh windfalls that have not yet been picked at by birds.

Once you have gathered your nuts, keep them in a dry, warm place but in their shells, so that the kernels don't dry out as well. You can use the nuts chopped or grated in salads, or with apple, raisins and raw oatmeal (muesli). Ground up in a blender, mixed with milk and chilled, they make a passable imitation of the Spanish drink *horchata* (properly made from the roots of the nutsedge, Cyperus esculentus). But hazelnuts are such a rich food that it seems wasteful not to use them occasionally as a protein substitute. Weight for weight, they contain fifty per cent more protein, seven times more fat and five times more carbohydrate than hens' eggs. What better way of cashing in on such a meaty hoard than the unjustly infamous nut cutlet?

To make hazelnut bread, grind a cupful of young nuts, and mix with the same amount of self-raising flour, half a cup of sugar and a little salt. Beat an egg with milk, and add it to the mixture, beating then kneading it until you have a stiff dough. Mould to a loaf shape, and bake in a medium oven for 50 minutes.

Hazel leaves were used in the fifteenth century to make 'noteye', a highly spiced pork stew. The leaves were ground together and mixed with ginger, saffron, sugar, salt and vinegar, before being added to minced pork

Nut cutlet

50 g (2 oz) oil
50 g (2 oz) flour
500 ml (1 pint) stock
75 g (3 oz) breadcrumbs
50 g (2 oz) grated hazelnuts
Milk or beaten egg for glazing
Salt and pepper

1 Mix the oil and flour in a saucepan. Add the stock and simmer for ten minutes, stirring all the time.
2 Add the breadcrumbs and grated hazelnuts. Season.
3 Cool the mixture and shape into cutlets.
4 Dip the cutlets into an egg and milk mixture, coat with breadcrumbs and fry in oil until brown.

Lime

Tilia europaea

Common in parks, by roadsides and in ornamental woods and copses. The lime is a tall tree, up to 45 m (150 ft) when it is allowed to grow naturally, with a smooth, dark brown trunk usually interrupted by bosses and side shoots. Flowers in July, a drooping cluster of heavily scented yellow blossoms. Leaves are large and heart-shaped, smooth above, paler below with a few tufts of fine white hairs.

The common lime is a cultivated hybrid between the two species of native wild lime, small-leaved (*Tilia cordata*) and large-leaved (*T. platyphyllos*), and it is now much commoner than both. It is one of the most beneficent of trees: its branches are a favourite site for mistletoe; its inner bark, bast, was used for making twine; its pale, close-grained timber is ideal for carving; its fragrant flowers make one of the best honeys. Limes are remarkable for the fact that they can, in flower, be tracked down by sound. In high summer their flowers are often so laden with bees that they can be heard 50 m (160 ft) away.

The leaves make a useful salad vegetable. When young they are thick, cooling, and very glutinous. Before they begin to roughen, they make a sandwich filling, between thin slices of new bread, with unsalted butter and just a sprinkling of lemon juice. Cut off the stalks and wash well, but otherwise put them between the bread as they come off the tree. Some aficionados enjoy them when they are sticky with the honeydew produced by aphid invasions in the summer.

In late June and July the yellow flowers of mature lime trees have a delicious honey-like fragrance, and make one of the very best teas of all wild flowers. It is popular in France, where it is sold under the name of *tilleul*.

Tilleul

Gather the flowers whilst they are in full bloom, in June or early July, and lay them out on trays or sheets of paper in a warm, well-ventilated room to dry. After two or three weeks they should have turned brittle and will be ready for use. Make tea from them in the usual way, experimenting with strengths, and serve like China tea, without milk.

Sloe, Blackthorn

Prunus spinosa

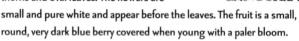

Widespread and abundant in woods and hedgerows throughout the British Isles, though thinning out in the north of Scotland. A stiff, dense shrub, up to 6 m (20 ft) high, with long thorns and oval leaves. The flowers are small and pure white and appear before the leaves. The fruit is a small, round, very dark blue berry covered when young with a paler bloom.

The sloe is one of the ancestors of cultivated plums. Crossed with the cherry plum (*Prunus cerasifera*), selected, crossed again, it eventually produced fruits as sweet and sumptuous as the Victoria plum. Yet the wild sloe is the tartest, most acid berry you will ever taste. Just one cautious bite into the green flesh will make the whole of the inside of your mouth creep. But a barrowload of sloe-stones was collected during the excavation of a Neolithic lake village at Glastonbury. Were they just used for dyeing? Or did our ancestors have hardier palates than us?

For all its potent acidity, the sloe is very far from being a useless fruit. It makes a clear, sprightly jelly, and that most agreeable of liqueurs, sloe gin.

Sloe gin

The best time to pick sloes for this drink is immediately after the first frost, which makes the skins softer and more permeable. Sloe gin made at this time will, providentially, just be ready in time for Christmas. Pick about a pound of the marble-sized berries (you will probably need a glove as the spines are stiff and sharp). If they have not been through a frost, pierce the skin of each one with a skewer, to help the gin and the juices get together more easily. Mix the sloes with a quarter of their weight of sugar, and half fill the bottles with this mixture. Pour gin into the bottles until they are nearly full, and seal tightly. Store for at least two months, and shake occasionally to help dissolve and disperse the sugar. The result is a brilliant, deep pink liqueur, sour-sweet and refreshing to taste, and demonstrably potent. Don't forget to eat the berries from the bottle, which will have quite lost their bitter edge, and soaked up a fair amount of the gin themselves. As an alternative, try replacing the gin in the recipe above with brandy or aquavit.

• •

Wild Cherry

Prunus avium

Widespread and frequent in hedgerows and woods, especially beech. A lofty tree, up to 30 m (100 ft) high, with shining, reddish-brown bark and an abundance of five-petalled white flowers in the spring.

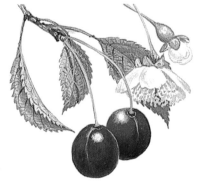

Leaves are alternate, oval, sharply toothed. The fruit is like a small, dark red, cultivated cherry.

The wild cherry is a beautiful tree in the springtime, and again in autumn when the leaves turn red. The fruit can be either sweet or bitter. It used to be sold occasionally in London on the branch.

These are the best fruits to use for cherry brandy. Put as many as you an find in a bottle with a couple of teaspoons of sugar, and top up with brandy. After three or four months you will have a treat waiting in your larder.

Bullace, Damsons and Wild Plums

Prunus species

The true bullace, Prunus domestica ssp. insititia, may be a scarce native of old hedgerows, but the majority of wild plums found in the countryside are either seeded from garden trees or are reverted orchard specimens. Fruit blue-black, brownish, or green-yellow, and usually midway in size between a sloe and a cultivated damson.

Wild plums are ripe from early October, and, unlike sloes, are usually just about sweet enough to eat raw. Otherwise they can be used like sloes, in jellies, gin, and autumn puddings (see p. 113).

Wild plums make excellent dark jams, and the French jam specialist Gisèle Tronche has pointed out how the addition of a little ground cumin seed and aniseed can improve conventional recipes. Alternatively try her late-autumn, wild fruit *humeur noir*, which she describes as having 'the colour of a good, healthy, black-tempered funk'.

Wild fruit jam

Crush together 800 g (2 lb) of stoned dark damsons and 200 g (8 oz) sugar, and leave overnight. Boil together 200 g (8 oz) of elderberries and 600 g (1½ lb) of blackberries for ten minutes. Add the damsons, another 600 g (1½ lb) of sugar, a tablespoon of cider vinegar and the juice of one lemon, and bring to the boil again. Cook for about an hour, until the desired consistency is reached. Pour into jars, leave to cool, and then seal.

• •

Rowan, Mountain-ash

Sorbus aucuparia

Widespread and common in dry woods and rocky places, especially on acid soils in the north and west of the British Isles. A small tree, up to 20 m (65 ft), with fairly smooth grey bark, toothed pinnate leaves, and umbels of small white flowers. Fruit: large clusters of small orange or red berries, August to November.

The rowan is a favourite municipal tree, and is planted in great numbers along the edges of residential highways, but you should not have too much trouble in finding wild specimens. Their clusters of brilliant orange fruits are unmistakable in almost every setting, against grey limestone in the uplands, or the deep evergreen of Scots pine on wintry heaths. Unless the birds have got there first, rowan berries can hang on the trees until January. They are best picked in October, when they have their full colour but have not yet become mushy.

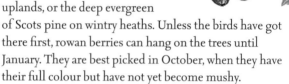

You should cut the clusters whole from the trees, trim off any excess stalk, and then make a jelly in the usual way (see p. 29), with the addition of a little chopped crab apple to provide the pectin. (You should be able to find crabs growing not far away from your rowans.)

The jelly is a deliciously dark orange, with a sharp, marmaladish flavour, and is perfect with game and lamb.

• •

Wild Service-tree

Sorbus torminalis

A relative of the rowan and the whitebeam, largely confined to ancient woods and hedgerows on limestone soils in the west and stiff clays in the Midlands and south. Up to 25 m (80 ft), a sign of ancient woodland. Leaves are alternate, deeply toothed, in pairs. Flowers are white branched clusters, May to June. Fruit is brown and speckled, 12–18 mm ($\frac{1}{2}$–$\frac{3}{4}$ inch).

The wild service-tree is one of the most local and retiring of our native trees, and knowledge of the fascinating history of its fruits has only recently been rediscovered.

The fruits, which appear in September, are round or pear-shaped and the size of small cherries. They are hard and bitter at first, but as autumn progresses they 'blet' – or go rotten – and become very sweet. The taste is unlike anything else which grows wild in this country, with hints of damson, prune, apricot, sultana and tamarind.

Remains of the berries have been found in prehistoric sites, and they must have been a boon before other sources of sugar were available. In areas where the tree was relatively widespread (e.g. the Weald of Kent) they continued to be a popular dessert fruit up to the beginning of the twentieth century. The fruits were gathered before they had bletted and strung up in clusters around a stick, which was hung up indoors, often by the hearth. They were picked off and eaten as they ripened, like sweets.

The tree is also known as the chequer tree, referring to the traditional pub name Chequers (the chequer board was the symbol for an inn or tavern in Roman times). The berries were used quite extensively in brewing.

Chequerberry beer

I have the house recipe for 'chequerberry beer' from the Chequers Inn at Smarden, Kent.

'Pick off in bunches in October. Hang on a string like onions (look like swarm of bees). Hang till ripe. Cut off close to berries. Put them in stone or glass jars. Put sugar on – 1 lb to 5 lb of berries. Shake up well. Keep airtight until juice comes to the top. The longer kept the better. Can add brandy. Drink. Then eat berries!'

Whitebeam

Sorbus aria

**Locally frequent in scrub and
copses in the south of England,
and popular as a suburban
roadside tree. Also a very striking
shrub, flashed with silver when the wind turns up the pale
undersides of the leaves.**

The bunched red berries are edible as soon as they begin to
'blet', like service berries. In the seventeenth century John
Evelyn recommended them in a concoction with new wine
and honey, though they are rather disappointing.

Juneberry

Amelanchier lamarckii

**An American shrub
naturalised in
woodlands in a few
areas of the south of
England, notably on
sandy soils in Sussex. Up to 10 m
(33 ft) high. Leaves alternate, oblong. Drifts of white
blossom in April and May. Fruit purplish-red/black,
10 mm ($^1/_2$ inch) with withered sepals, in June.**

The purplish-red berries rarely form in this country, but they
are sweet to taste, and can be eaten uncooked or made into
pies. In America they are sometimes canned for winter use.

Medlar

Mespilus germanica

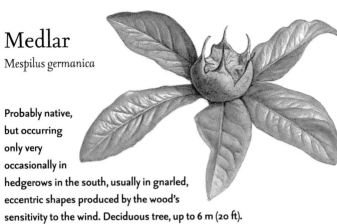

Probably native, but occurring only very occasionally in hedgerows in the south, usually in gnarled, eccentric shapes produced by the wood's sensitivity to the wind. Deciduous tree, up to 6 m (20 ft). Leaves alternate, crinkled, white hairs beneath. Flowers have five white petals with longer green sepals, May to June. Fruit like a giant brown rosehip, with the five-tailed calyx protruding from the head of the fruit like a crown.

The curious fact about the medlar is that its fruits need to be half-rotten – or 'bletted' – before they are edible. This seems to be a result of our climate not being warm enough to ripen the fruits, for in Mediterranean regions, where the tree is more widespread, the young fruit can be eaten straight off the tree. Here it stays rock-hard until mid-winter.

When the fruits are fully bletted, usually not before the November frosts, the brown flesh can be scraped out of the skin and eaten with cream and sugar. The fruits can also be baked whole, like apples, or made into jelly.

* * * * *

Hawthorn, May-tree

Crataegus monogyna

Widespread and abundant on heaths, downs, hedges, scrubland, light woods and all open land. Small tree or large shrub, up to 6 m

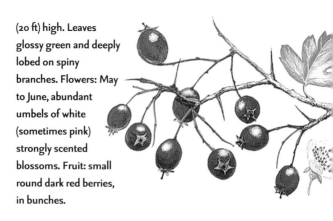

(20 ft) high. Leaves glossy green and deeply lobed on spiny branches. Flowers: May to June, abundant umbels of white (sometimes pink) strongly scented blossoms. Fruit: small round dark red berries, in bunches.

The young April leaves – traditionally called bread and cheese by children in England – have a pleasantly nutty taste. Eat them straight from the tree or use them in sandwiches, or in any of the recipes for wild spring greens. They also blend well with potatoes and almost any kind of nuts. A sauce for spring lamb can be made by chopping the leaves with other early wild greens, such as garlic mustard and sorrel, and dressing with vinegar and brown sugar, as with a mint sauce. The leaf buds can be picked much earlier in the year, though it takes an age to gather any quantity, and they tend to fall apart anyway. Dorothy Hartley has a splendid recipe for a spring pudding which makes use of the buds, for those with the patience to collect large numbers of them.

Hawthorn berries (haws) are perhaps the most abundant berry of all in the autumn. Almost every hawthorn bush is festooned with small bunches of the round, dark-red berries, looking rather like spherical rosehips. When fully ripe they taste a little like avocado pear. They make a moderate jelly, but being a dry fruit need long simmering with a few crab apples to bring out all the juices and provide the necessary pectin. Otherwise the jelly will be sticky or rubbery. It is a good accompaniment to cream cheese.

Hawthorn spring pudding
(Dorothy Hartley)

Make a light suet crust, well seasoned, and roll it out thinly and as long in shape as possible. Cover the surface with the young leaves, and push them slightly into the suet. Take some rashers of bacon, cut into fine strips and lay them across the leaves. Moisten the edges of the dough and roll it up tightly, sealing the edges as you go. Tie in a cloth and steam for at least an hour. Cut it in thick slices like a Swiss roll, and serve with gravy.

Elder
Sambucus nigra

Widespread and common in woods, hedgerows and waste places. A tall, fast-growing shrub, up to 10 m (33 ft), with a corky bark, white pith in the heart of the branches, and a scaly surface to the young twigs. Leaves usually in groups of five; large, dark green and slightly toothed. Flowers are umbels of numerous tiny creamy-white flowers, June to July. Fruits are clusters of small, reddish-black berries, August to October.

To see the mangy, decaying skeletons of elders in the winter you would not think the bush was any use to man or beast. Nor would the acrid stench of the young leaves in spring change your opinion. But by the end of June the whole shrub is covered with great sprays of sweet-smelling flowers, for which there are probably more uses than any other single species of blossom. Even in orthodox medicine they have an acknowledged role as an ingredient in skin ointments and eye-lotions.

Elderflowers can be munched straight off the branch on a hot summer's day, and taste as frothy as a glass of ice-cream soda. Something even closer to that drink can be made by putting a bunch of elderflowers in a jug with boiling water, straining the liquid off when cool, and sweetening.

Cut the elderflower clusters whole, with about 5 cm (2 inches) of stem attached to them. Always check that they are free of insects, and discard any that are badly infested. The odd grub or two can be removed by hand. But never wash the flowers, as this will remove much of the fragrance. The young buds can be pickled or added to salads. The flowers themselves, separated from the stalks, make what is indisputably the best sparkling wine besides champagne. But one of the most famous recipes for elderflowers is the preserve they make with gooseberries.

Elderflower and gooseberry preserve

To make the preserve, trim off as much of the rather bitter stalk as you can, and have ready four flower heads for each 500 g (1 lb) of gooseberries. Top, tail and wash the gooseberries in the usual way, and put them into a pan with 500 ml (1 pint) of water for every 500 g of fruit. Simmer for half an hour, mashing the fruit to a pulp as you do. Add 500 g of sugar for each 500 g of fruit, stir rapidly until dissolved, and bring to the boil. Then add the elder-flowers, tied in muslin, and boil rapidly until the setting point is reached. Remove the flowers and pot in the usual way. (See p. 29 for a few extra notes on jams and jellies generally.) The flavour is quite transformed from that of plain gooseberry jam, and reminiscent of Muscat grapes. It is good with ice-cream and other sweets.

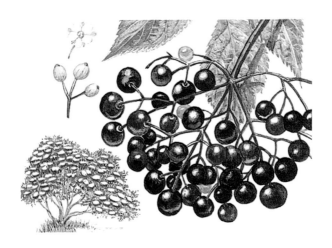

Elderflower fritters

A perfect and delicately flavoured finish to a summer meal.

4 tablespoons flour
1 egg
1½ cupfuls water
Elderflower heads
(retain short stalks for dipping)
Oil for frying
Fresh mint
Sugar for dusting

1 Make up the batter with the flour, egg and water.
2 Hold the flower-head by the stalk and dip into the batter.
3 Shake off any excess batter, then plunge into hot oil and deep-fry until golden-brown.
4 Trim off the excess stalk and serve with sugar and mint and lemon.

Elderflower cordial

This cordial will keep for six months, or you can freeze it as ice cubes or in plastic bottles (leaving room for expansion).

1 lemon
25 g (1 oz) citric acid
1 kg (2 lb) sugar
10 elderflower heads
750 ml (1½ pints) water

1 Put the sugar in a large bowl and pour on the boiling water. Stir to dissolve.
2 Grate the lemon rind, and slice the fruit.
3 Add the grated lemon rind, lemon slices, citric acid and flower-heads to the water.
4 Leave for 24 hours, stirring occasionally.
5 Sieve through muslin, pour into clean bottles and seal with screw-top caps.

Elderberries are useful as additions to a number of cooked recipes, in which any unpleasant aftertaste completely disappears.

The berries are ripe when the clusters begin to turn upside down. Gather the clusters whole by cutting them from the stems, picking only those where the very juicy berries have not started to wrinkle or melt. Wash them well, and strip them from the stalks with a fork. They are good added whole to apple pies, or added as a make-weight to blackberry jelly. (Both berries are on the bush at the same time, so if you are making this they can be gathered straight into the same basket.)

My favourite elderberry recipe is for Pontack sauce, a relic from those days when every retired military gentleman carried his patent sauce as an indispensable part of his luggage.

Pontack sauce

There are any number of variants of Pontack sauce, particularly from the traditional hunting country in the Midlands. This one from Leicestershire probably used claret instead of vinegar in the original (Pontack's was owned by Château Haut-Brion).

500 ml (1 pint) boiling vinegar (or claret)
500 ml (1 pint) elderberries
1 teaspoon salt
1 blade mace
40 peppercorns
12 cloves
1 onion, finely chopped
1/2 teaspoon ginger

1 Pour the vinegar (or claret) over the elderberries in a stone jar or casserole dish. Cover and allow to stand overnight in an oven at very low heat.
2 Next day pour off the liquid, put it in a saucepan with the salt, mace, peppercorns, cloves, onion and ginger.
3 Boil for 10 minutes and then bottle securely with the spices.

The sauce was reputedly meant to be kept for seven years before use. My patience ran out after seven days, but having made rather a large bottle, I can report a distinct improvement in richness after the first few years! It has a fine fruity taste, a little like a thick punch, and is especially good with liver.

Herbaceous plants

Maidenhair Fern
Adiantum capillus-veneris

A rare and delicate fern which grows on sheltered limestone cliffs in a few localities in the west.

In the eighteenth and nineteenth centuries maidenhair fern was used as a garnish to sweet dishes. Later it formed the basis of capillaire, which was a popular flavouring in the late nineteenth century. The fern (imported from Iceland) was simmered in water for several hours, and the liquid made into a thick syrup with sugar and orange-water. Capillaire was mixed with fruit juice and water to form soft drinks.

Oregon-grape
Mahonia aquifolium

A member of the barberry family, originally from North America and naturalised in open woodland and game coverts. An evergreen shrub, up to 150 cm (5 ft) high. Leaves holly-like, with sharp spines. Flowers yellow and fragrant. The dark, white-bloomed berries form in bunches like miniature grapes.

Oregon-grapes are planted to provide cover and food for pheasants. The berries can be eaten raw, though they are rather acid, and are best made into a jelly.

Common Poppy, Field Poppy

Papaver rhoeas

Widespread and abundant in arable fields and by roadsides. Becomes scarcer in Wales, northwest England and northern Scotland. Flowers June to October, deep scarlet, floppy petals at the top of a thin, hairy stalk, 30–60 cm (1–2 ft) high. The seed-pods are hairless, and flat-topped like an inverted cone.

Poppies and cornfields have long been associated in our consciousness, from the Roman goddess Ceres, who was depicted with a bunch of poppies in one hand, to Monet's atmospheric, sun-drenched landscapes. The plant probably arrived in Britain with the first Neolithic settlers, and it thrived in the countryside. Aggressive use of herbicides virtually eliminated the poppy from our fields after the Second World War, and the plant became confined to roadsides and waste places. More recently, however, changes in farming practices and a revival of interest in the flower have heralded its return to our landscape.

It was once believed that smelling poppies gave you a headache, and that staring at them for too long made you go blind. Superstition about the supposed poisonousness of the flower still persist, notably the belief that the seed heads contain opium. In fact no parts of the common field poppy are narcotic, least of all the dry seeds. It is the Asian species *Papaver somniferum* from which opium is derived, by the cutting and tapping of the juice from the unripe seed heads. Yet the dry ripe seeds of the opium poppy are entirely edible, and indeed are the poppy seeds of commerce, used extensively in baking. Common poppy seeds make an acceptable, though less flavoursome, substitute.

The seed heads start to dry in September, and are ready for picking when they are grey-brown in colour, and have a number of small holes just below the edge of the flat top. These are vents through which the seeds normally escape, and the seed in ripe heads can be readily shaken out of the holes.

Pick a handful of these heads and put them straight into a paper bag. Remove the seeds by inverting the heads and shaking them into the bag. Any that cling on to their contents are not really ripe.

Poppy seeds are slate grey in colour and have an elusive taste. They are extensively used in European and Middle Eastern cookery, particularly for sprinkling on bread, rolls, cakes and biscuits. But they also go well with honey as a dressing for fruit, and with noodles and macaroni.

Stinging Nettle
Urtica dioica

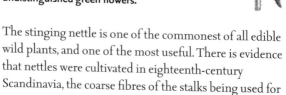

Widespread and abundant in almost every sort of environment, particularly waste and cultivated ground, wet woods, hedgebanks, river valleys. A coarse, upright plant, growing up to 120 cm (4 ft) high, covered with stinging hairs. Leaves toothed and heart-shaped. Flowers June to September, thin catkins of tiny, undistinguished green flowers.

The stinging nettle is one of the commonest of all edible wild plants, and one of the most useful. There is evidence that nettles were cultivated in eighteenth-century Scandinavia, the coarse fibres of the stalks being used for cloth as well as the leaves for food. Samuel Pepys enjoyed a nettle 'porridge' on 25 February 1661, though he gives no details of the dish. Sir Walter Scott has the old gardener in Rob Roy raising nettles under glass as 'early spring kail'. And in the Second World War hundreds of tons were gathered annually in Great Britain for the extraction of chlorophyll, and to make dyes for camouflage nets.

Nettles and people are plainly old companions. Wherever the soil has been enriched by human settlement – be it boneyards or back gardens – there will be nettles. Because they take up nutrients very slowly, nettles can be astonishingly persistent on such sites. In woods in the Salisbury area they are still flourishing on the buried refuse of Roman-British villages abandoned 1,600 years ago.

The striking ability of nettles to make use of minerals and nitrogen in enriched soils gives them a high ranking in nutrition tables. They have high levels of vitamins A and C, 2.3 per cent by weight of iron, and a remarkable 5.5 per cent of protein.

Nettles should not be picked for eating after the beginning of June. In high summer the leaves become coarse in texture, unpleasantly bitter in taste and decidedly laxative. The best time of all for them is when the young shoots are no more than about 20 centimetres high. Pick these shoots whole or, if you are gathering later in the year, just the tops and the young pale green leaves. It is as well to use gloves whilst doing this, even if you do have a Spartan belief in the protection of the firm grasp.

Before cooking your nettles remove the tougher stems and wash well. They can be used in a number of ways. As a straight vegetable they should be boiled gently in a closed pan for about four minutes, in no more water than adheres to the leaves after washing. Strain off the water well, add a large knob of butter and plenty of seasoning (and perhaps some chopped onion), and simmer for a further five minutes, turning and mashing all the while. The resulting purée is interestingly fluffy in texture, but rather insipid – don't expect it to taste like spinach, as is sometimes suggested. For my money nettles are better used as additions to other dishes, or as the basis for nettle soup, than as vegetables in their own right.

Nettle purée can be spread on toast and served with a poached egg on top, or mixed into balls with oatmeal and fried in bacon fat as a kind of rissole. Another splendid recipe is for nettle haggis. The nettle purée is mixed with leeks and cabbage, freshly fried bacon and partially cooked oatmeal (or rice or barley), the whole boiled for an hour or so in a muslin bag, and served with gravy. More modern recipes include deep-frying the leaves to the consistency of green crisps. Young nettle leaves have also been made into beer and used as the basis for a herbal tea.

Note: to be caught eating nettles will cause more consternation amongst your friends than the munching of any number of other more dubious plants. Reassure them that the chemicals responsible for the sting are quite destroyed by cooking – and offer them a taste.

Nettle soup

4 large handfuls of nettle tops
1 large onion
50 g (2 oz) butter
2 potatoes
1 litre (2 pints) vegetable stock
1 tablespoon crème fraîche
Seasoning, including grated nutmeg

1 Strip the nettles from the thicker stalks, and wash.
2 Melt the butter and simmer the chopped onion in it until golden.
3 Add the nettles (or an equivalent amount of nettle

purée) and the chopped potatoes, and cook for
2–3 minutes.

4 Add the stock, and simmer for 20 minutes, using a
wooden spoon from time to time to crush the
potatoes.

5 Add the seasoning, plus a little grated nutmeg, and
serve with a swirl of crème fraîche.

6 If you prefer a smoother soup, put the mixture
through a liquidiser before serving. Reheat, and add
seasoning and crème fraîche.

Bog-myrtle, Sweet Gale
Myrica gale

**Locally common in bogs, marshes and wet
heaths, mainly in Scotland, Ireland, north Wales
and the northwest of England. Flowers April to
May. A deciduous shrub, 60–180 cm (2–6 ft) high
with red and orange (female and male) catkins on
separate plants. These flowers appear in April or
May, before the leaves, which are grey-green,
narrow, toothed, on shiny reddish twigs.**

Before the extensive draining of fen and
wetlands that began in the sixteenth century,
bog-myrtle, or sweet gale, must have been a
much more widespread plant. Now it is only locally
common in wet, acid heathland and moors, mainly in the
north and west, though some small, local populations do
occur in southern England. Where it does appear, its leaves
and flowers can scent the whole area with their delightfully
sweet, resinous smell.

Gale was traditionally used for the flavouring of beer, before hops were taken into service in this country. There is evidence that this drink was being brewed in Anglo-Saxon times, and the isolated patches of sweet gale which grow around old monasteries and other early settlements suggest that it was occasionally taken into cultivation, outside its natural habitats.

The brewing recipe is rather elaborate, so experiment with sweet gale as a herb, and use it to flavour existing drinks. Its warm aroma – with hints of balsam, cloves and pine resin – will give a retsina-like tang to wine, if sprigs of bog-myrtle are steeped in the wine (in re-sealed bottles) for a month. The leaves are also good as a stuffing for roast chicken.

· ·

Hottentot-fig

Carpobrotus edulis

Trailing branched perennial with fleshy leaves, introduced from South Africa. Yellow, pink or magenta flowers with yellow stamens. Fleshy fruit appears May to July. Found on cliffs, particularly in Devon and Cornwall.

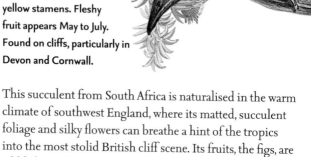

This succulent from South Africa is naturalised in the warm climate of southwest England, where its matted, succulent foliage and silky flowers can breathe a hint of the tropics into the most stolid British cliff scene. Its fruits, the figs, are edible but rather tangy.

Fat-hen

Chenopodium album

Common in cultivated and waste ground throughout Britain. An undistinguished plant, 20–150 cm (8–60 inches) tall, with stiff upright stems and diamond-shaped greyish-green leaves. Flowers June to September, pale green, minute and bunched into spikes.

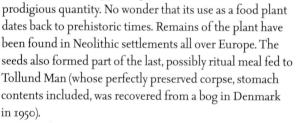

Fat-hen is one of those plants that thrive in the company of humans. Prepare a manure heap in your garden and fat-hen will in all likelihood begin to grow there within a few months. It is one of the very first plants to colonise ground that has been disturbed by roadworks or house-building, its stiff, mealy spikes often appearing in prodigious quantity. No wonder that its use as a food plant dates back to prehistoric times. Remains of the plant have been found in Neolithic settlements all over Europe. The seeds also formed part of the last, possibly ritual meal fed to Tollund Man (whose perfectly preserved corpse, stomach contents included, was recovered from a bog in Denmark in 1950).

In Anglo-Saxon times the plant was apparently of sufficient importance to have villages named after it. As *melde* it is thought to have given its name to Melbourn in Cambridgeshire and Milden in Suffolk. The introduction of spinach, a domesticated relative, largely put an end to the use of the plant, but its leaves continued to be eaten in Ireland and the Scottish islands for a long while, and in many parts of Europe during the famine conditions of the

Second World War. We now know that early people were lucky in their choice of fat-hen as a staple vegetable, for it contains more iron and protein than either cabbage or spinach, and more vitamin B1 and calcium than raw cabbage.

The whole plant can be eaten raw, but it is probably best prepared and cooked in the same way as spinach, as a green vegetable, or in soups. It is pleasantly tangy, like young kale or broccoli.

• •

Good-King-Henry

Chenopodium bonus-henricus

Widespread but rather local by roadsides and in cultivated ground; less common in Wales, Scotland, Ireland and the southwest. A medium perennial, often reddish, up to 80 cm (2–3 ft). Leaves triangular or spear-shaped, almost untoothed. Flowers in spikes, May to August.

The curious name has nothing to do with Henry VIII or any other king. It is a corruption of 'Good Henry', an elfin figure from Saxon folklore whose name was applied to this plant to distinguish it from 'Bad Henry', the poisonous annual mercury (Mercurialis annua) or dog's mercury (see p. 125), with which it sometimes grows but which it in no way resembles.

Good-King-Henry is another food plant of great antiquity, the remains of which have been found in

Neolithic encampments. It is a native of the Mediterranean, and its seeds may have been brought over as weeds by the first farmers over 5,000 years ago. In medieval and Elizabethan times it was occasionally taken into cultivation, and it has lately come back into popularity (and commerce) as a herb-garden species.

Good-King-Henry is a perennial, which means that leaves can be picked from it continuously, as from an everlasting spinach. The leaves can be cooked as a spinach, and the young shoots like asparagus, if they are picked in the spring when they are not more than 20 cm (8 inches) high. Strip off the larger leaves, bind the shoots in small bundles, then simmer in water for no more than five minutes and serve with melted butter.

Sea-purslane

Atriplex portulacoides

Common on salt marshes in the south and east of England. Flowers July to October.

The oval, fleshy leaves of this maritime plant make a succulent addition to salads. They can also be stir-fried with fish or meat.

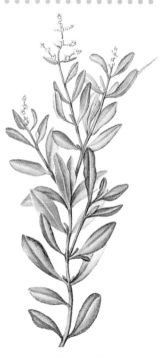

Common Orache

Atriplex patula

Widespread and abundant throughout the British Isles, on bare and waste ground. Flowers July to September.

Young leaves and shoots may be used as a substitute for spinach.

Spear-leaved Orache

Atriplex prostrata

Frequent throughout the British Isles, especially near the sea. Flowers July to September.

Another species of orache that can be used as a spinach-substitute.

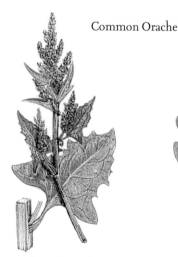

Common Orache

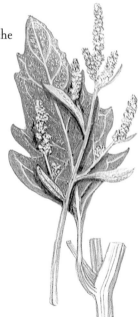

Spear-leaved Orache

Sea Beet,
Wild Spinach
Beta vulgaris ssp. maritima

Common on banks and shingle by the sea, except in Scotland. Perennial, up to 90 cm (3 ft) high, with shiny, fleshy leaves. Flowers June to September, tiny green blossoms in long leafy spikes.

One of the happy exceptions to the small-leaved tendency among wild vegetables. Some of the bottom leaves of the sea beet can grow as large and as heavy as those of any cultivated spinach, and creak like parchment when you touch them.

The wild plant is one of the ancestors of our cultivated beets, from mangelwurzels through to chards and spinach-beet. Cultivation began at least 2,000 years ago in the Middle East, and was mostly directed towards filling out the long tap root into the forms we now pickle, feed to cattle or convert to sugar. If you look closely at some of the wild specimens you will occasionally find a red-veined individual that is from the strain that was developed into the beetroot.

The leaves have been changed little by cultivation, except to lose some of their powerful tannin-and-iron flavour. You can pick them between April and October – big, fleshy ones from the base of the plant and thinner, spear-shaped ones near the head. Try and strip the larger leaves from their central spine as you pick them: it will save much time during preparation for cooking.

Always take special care in washing wild spinach leaves (especially if they have been picked near public footpaths, where their bushy clumps can be targets for perambulating dogs). Remove also the miscellaneous herbage you will inevitably have grubbed up whilst picking the leaves, and the more substantial stems.

Sea beet can be used in identical ways to garden spinach. The small leaves which grow on specimens very close to the sea are tender and succulent, often as much as a millimetre thick, and are ideal for salads. The larger ones should be steamed, or boiled briskly in a large saucepan with no more than a sprinkle of water at the bottom. Leave the lid on for a few minutes, and at intervals chop and press down the leaves. When the vegetable has changed colour to a very dark green, remove the lid altogether and simmer for a further two or three minutes to boil off some of the remaining water, then transfer to a colander and press out as much liquid as possible (saving it for stock or gravy). Return the greens to the saucepan, and toss over a low heat with a knob of butter. The taste is a good deal tangier than cultivated spinach, and good additions are diced tomatoes and grated nuts.

Spinach tart

This seventeenth-century tart is one of the most intriguing recipes I know for sea beet. Boil the leaves in the usual way, and chop them up with a few hard-boiled egg yolks. Set into a pastry tart case, and pour on a sauce made of melted sugar, raisins and a touch of cinnamon. Bake in a moderate oven for about half an hour.

Marsh Samphire, Glasswort

Salicornia species

Common and often abundant on salt marshes round most British coasts. Succulent annuals, varying from single unbranched stems to thick stubby bushes up to 30 cm (1 ft) tall. The stems are plump, shiny and jointed. Flowers minute, and only really visible as one or two white to red stamens growing out of the junctions in the stems, August to September.

Samphire has a liking for muddy situations, and grows in such abundance on some salt marshes that a communal forage is the most sensible and agreeable way to harvest it. You go out at low tide, with buckets and wellingtons, through the sea-aster and wormwood in the rough ground at the edge of the saltings, on to the tidal reaches where the crop grows. This is a world crisscrossed by deep and hidden creeks, by which you will be tripped, cut off and plastered up to the thigh with glistening wet mud. In these creeks the samphire grows tall and bushy, like an amiable maritime cactus.

On the poorer, sandier flats the plants are smaller, and they tend to grow as single shoots not more than 15 cm (6 inches) high. Yet they make up for this in sheer numbers. Often a bed can completely carpet several acres of marsh, and look as though it could be cut with a lawnmower. But there are no short cuts. Traditionally, samphire was gathered by pulling up by the roots. This is now illegal, so there is no escaping half an hour in a stooping position, snipping the stems individually with a sharp knife or pair of scissors. But then hunched up and grubbing about in the mud is the only true way to appreciate the delights of samphire gathering.

Collect the stems into a bucket, basket or best of all a string bag, and rinse the bunch roughly in sea water to remove the worst of the mud before taking the crop home. When you have got your samphire home, wash it well and remove the pieces of seaweed that will inevitably be stuck to some of the plants. But never leave samphire to stand in water for more than a few minutes. Its succulence is due to salt water stored by the plant, and the salt will quickly be sucked out into the fresh water, causing the plants to become limp and prone to decay. If you wish to keep it for a day or two before eating, dry it well and store, unwrapped, in the fridge.

The young shoots, picked in June or July, make a crisp and tangy salad vegetable. Try chewing some sprigs straight from the marsh. They are very refreshing in spite of their salty taste. To cook them, boil or steam in a little water for 8–10 minutes, drain and serve with melted butter. Eat by holding the stem at the base, dipping in the butter and sliding the stems between the teeth, to draw the flesh off the tough central spine. Samphire prepared like this can be served either as an asparagus-like starter or as a vegetable with fish, poultry or lamb.

A traditional way with samphire is to pickle it. In recent years I have found pickled samphire being offered as a bar-top nibble in north Norfolk pubs, and there are signs that the plant is becoming more popular. Samphire is also appearing increasingly on the menus of metropolitan restaurants, though sometimes only as a garnish, and often imported from the Continent.

Pickled samphire

This was once done by filling jars with the chopped shoots, covering with spiced vinegar, and placing in a baker's oven as it cooled off over the weekend. I would imagine that the result of 48 hours' simmering would be on the sloppy side, to say the least. To maintain the crisp texture of the plant and at least some of its brilliant green colour it is best to do no more than put it under cold pickling vinegar

Pigweed, Common Amaranth
Amaranthus retroflexus

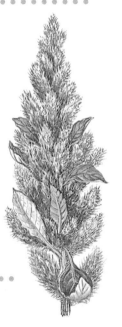

A curious casual of waste and cultivated ground, with dense spikes of dry, greenish flowers.

The plant originated in America and was much used by the indigenous people. The leaves, boiled, made a mild green vegetable, and the black seeds were ground into flour.

Chickweed
Stellaria media

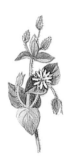

Widespread and abundant throughout the British Isles in gardens and disturbed ground. A weak plant which tends to straggle and creep before it has reached any height. It has single lines of fine hairs up alternate sides of the stem. Leaves oval, bright green and soft. Flowers throughout the year, a tiny, white, star-like flower, with five deeply divided petals.

Chickweed is generally regarded as a bane in gardens. Yet it is one of the most deliciously tender of all wild vegetables, with a taste reminiscent of cornsalad or a mild lettuce. The Elizabethan herbalist John Gerard prescribed it for 'little birdes in cadges ... when they loath their meate'. But even in his time it was cooked as a green vegetable, and later hawked around city streets by itinerant vegetable sellers. Chickweed is one of the earliest wild vegetables to come into leaf, and it is a good base for winter, or early spring, salads.

Next time you are weeding the garden, try saving the chickweed instead of composting it. Those without gardens should be able to find some by any field edge, even in the winter months. The leaves are too small to be picked individually, so strip bunches of the whole plant, or choose the younger, greener sprigs and cut with scissors. The stems are just as tender to eat as the leaves.

The texture and mild taste of chickweed is probably best appreciated in a salad. Try mixing the young shoots with hairy bitter-cress (for a hint of pepperiness), winter-cress and cow parsley, and dress with a light, sharp dressing made from lemon juice and sunflower oil.

Cooked chickweed

Wash the sprigs well, and put into a saucepan without any additional water. Add a knob of butter or a spoonful of oil, some chopped spring onions and seasoning. Simmer briefly for no more than two minutes – any longer and both taste and texture will go and you will be left with something resembling strands of green string. Finish off with a dash of lemon juice or a sprinkling of grated nutmeg.

Bladder Campion

Silene vulgaris

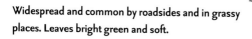

Widespread and common by roadsides and in grassy places. Leaves bright green and soft.

The young shoots and leaves can be used like chickweed, and added to spring salads or cooked as greens.

• •

Bistort

Persicaria bistorta

Widespread and locally common in wet, hilly pastures throughout the British Isles, except the south. Leaves oblong or arrow-shaped on long stalks. Flowers June to August, pink spikes topping off a straight, hairless stem about 60 cm (2 ft) high.

In the early spring of 1971 an advertisement in the personal columns of *The Times* invited entrants for the first World Dock Pudding Championship, to be held in the Calder Valley in West Yorkshire. In parts of northern England there was a tradition of making Easter puddings – 'dock puddings' – from bistort leaves and various combinations of oatmeal, egg and other green herbs. Like many local customs, the making of dock or ledger pudding had declined in the twentieth century, but the 1960s and 1970s saw a revival, and there were over fifty competitors from this one valley for the first world championship. The competition is still held annually in the town of Mytholmroyd, with competitors required to follow a basic recipe including bistort leaves, chopped nettles, onions and oatmeal, all fried in bacon fat.

Bistort is a plant of damp upland meadows, out of the range of nibbling sheep (though one Calder Valley man claimed that the best plants grew on his granddad's grave on Sowerby Top). It usually appears as a basic ingredient of Easter pudding, though quite why bistort should have been singled out as the vital ingredient in the sheep-grazing country of the north Pennines is hard to say. It can certainly be locally plentiful in damp hill pastures, and the leaves can be quite fleshy by Easter – but just as important may be the fact that bistort leaves have a comparatively mild taste, unlike some of the other customary ingredients of spring puddings. Many of the plant's local names refer to its function in this pudding, from Passion dock (from Passion-tide, the last two weeks of Lent, which was the proper time for eating this rather scant dish) to Easter giant, a contraction of Easter mangiant (from the French *manger*, to eat).

Dock pudding

There is an enormous variety of different recipes for dock pudding, most of them originating in the Lake District. This one is based on a recipe from Carlisle.

1 handful of bistort leaves
1 tablespoon each of the leaves of nettles, cabbage (or young leaves and shoots from Brussels sprouts) and dandelion, sorrel or dock
3 leeks
2 black currant leaves
1 cup cooked pearl barley
3 eggs
Oatmeal for binding and/or coating
Salt and pepper to taste, Oil or bacon fat

1 Chop the bistort, leeks and other greens roughly and blanch in boiling water for a few minutes.

2 Mix with the pearl barley, seasoning and two of the eggs, hard-boiled and chopped, and the other egg, beaten. Bind the mixture with a little oatmeal.

3 Either put the mixture in a pudding basin and boil for ten minutes, or form into balls, coat in oatmeal, and fry in oil or bacon fat.

Redshank

Persicaria maculosa

Widespread and common throughout the British Isles in damp, shady places, near ditches, etc. Flowers June to October.

Leaves are rather insipid, but they can be used in mixed greens, or in the dock pudding mix (see above).

Common Sorrel

Rumex acetosa

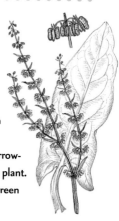

Widespread and common in grassland, meadows, heathland and roadsides, especially on acid soils, throughout the British Isles. An erect perennial, 10–120 cm (4–48 inches) high. Leaves arrow-shaped and clasping the stem near the top of the plant. Flowers May to August, spikes of small red and green flowers on a smooth stem.

Sorrel is one of the very first green plants to appear in the spring. The leaves can often be picked as early as February, when other greenstuffs are scarce. In parts of the north and the Midlands, sorrel was used as a substitute for apple in tarts and turnovers, during the fruit off-season between the last apples in March and the first gooseberries. Sorrel's plum-skin sharpness can make it an interesting stand-in for fruit in other dishes.

Sorrel makes a good lemony addition to salads throughout the spring and summer, especially if you cut or tear the strips across the grain (what the French refer to as chiffonade). They are marvellously cool and sharp when raw, like young plum skins, but perhaps too acid for some palates.

In Gerard's time the leaves were boiled and eaten, or made into a green sauce for fish. For this they were pulped raw and mixed with sugar and vinegar. Dorothy Hartley describes a late seventeenth-century recipe for the sauce, in which bread, apple, sugar and vinegar are boiled together until soft, then mixed, still hot, with sorrel purée. The mixture is then strained, yielding a thick green juice with a strong pungent taste.

In France sorrel is used in an enormous variety of dishes. The chopped leaves are added to give a sharp flavour to heavy soups of potato, lentil and haricot bean. The cooked purée is added to omelettes, or, like the sauce, served as an accompaniment to veal or fish dishes.

Sorrel soup

To make a rich sorrel soup, chop 500 g (1 lb) of the leaves with a large onion and a sprig of rosemary. Mix well with one tablespoon of flour and simmer the mixture in 75 g (3 oz) of butter for about ten minutes, stirring well all the time. Add 2 litres (4 pints) of boiling water, two tablespoons of breadcrumbs and seasoning. Simmer for one hour. When ready, take off the boil and just before serving stir in a well-beaten mixture of two egg yolks and 150 ml (¼ pint) of yoghurt.

Curled Dock

Rumex crispus

The most widespread of all our docks, growing as happily in seaside shingle as in suburban field edges.

The crinkly leaves, which can grow up to 30 cm (1 ft) long, are bitter, but have been used as a vegetable in the United States. The leaves are gathered very young and cooked with bacon or ham and a little vinegar. The leaves of our commonest dock, the broad-leaved dock (*Rumex obtusifolius*), have been used in the same way, though they are even more bitter.

Parents can pick a leaf or two of dock and crumple them up to rub into the skin of a small child who has been stung by a nettle. The miraculous alleviation of the pain is probably entirely psychological; but the confidence-trick is as valuable as the notions of tooth-fairies and Father Christmas, and should be perpetuated stoutly.

Monk's-rhubarb

Rumex pseudoalpinus

An uncommon species of dock, with large heart-shaped leaves.

Monk's-rhubarb was introduced as a pot-herb in the Middle Ages, and in the parts of Scotland and the north of England, where it still grows, it is rarely found far from houses.

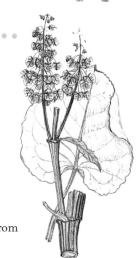

Common Mallow

Malva sylvestris

Widespread and abundant on banks, roadsides and waste places, especially near the sea. Rather less common in Scotland. The plant is coarse, bushy and often straggly, 20–100 cm (8–40 inches) high, and carries crinkly, ivy-shaped leaves which are slightly clammy to touch when young. Flowers from June to October, five-petalled, purplish blossoms up to 4 cm (2 inches) across.

Mallow blooms late into the autumn, and its flowers have a strange, artificial elegance that is unexpected in such an obviously hardy wayside weed. The mauve petals are arched like some porcelain decoration, and veined with deep purple streaks.

The leaves stay green and fresh almost all the year, but are best picked in the summer months, when they can be stretched like films of gelatine. Always wash the leaves well and discard any that have developed a brownish rust, or are embedded with tiny black insect eggs.

Mallow leaves can be cooked as a spinach, but they are extremely glutinous, and a more attractive way of using them is to make them into soup. In Arab countries, notably Egypt, the leaves of a similar species are the basis of the famous soup, *melokhia*.

Common mallow is also known for its small, round seeds, called 'cheeses' (from their taste, which is mildly nutty). Children in country districts still pick and eat these, though they're such a diminutive mouthful that their taste and texture are hardly noticeable. Some experimenters have found that modern children are more attracted by the leaves, deep-fried in hot oil until they resemble a wafer-thin green crisp!

Melokhia

A fairly authentic version of the Egyptian soup.
The melokhia can be served on its own, or with boiled
rice, or with pieces of cooked meat and vegetables.

500 g (1 lb) young mallow leaves
1 litre (2 pints) chicken stock
2 cloves garlic
Oil for frying
1 dessertspoon ground coriander
Pinch cayenne pepper, salt to taste

1 Remove the stalks from the mallow leaves, wash
well, and chop very small or purée in a blender.
2 Boil the leaves in the chicken stock for ten minutes.
3 In a separate pan, prepare a garlic sauce by frying
the crushed garlic in a little oil until golden brown,
adding the coriander, cayenne pepper and some salt,
and mixing to a paste in the hot pan.
4 Add this paste to the soup, cover the saucepan
tightly and simmer for 2–3 minutes, stirring
occasionally to prevent the leaves falling to the
bottom.

● ●

Marsh-mallow

Althaea officinalis

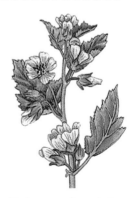

A tall perennial, 1.5–2m (5–6 ft), which
grows near salt water in southern and
eastern England. Soft-branched clumps
with velvety pink flowers between July
and September.

The plant that gave the sweet its name. Today marshmallow is made from starch, gelatine and sugar. But it was once produced from the roots of *Althaea officinalis*, which contain not only their own starch, but also albumen, a crystallisable sugar, a fixed oil and a good deal of gelatinous matter. They were gathered by fishermen's wives in the dykes and salt marshes of the east coast.

• •

Sweet Violet
Viola odorata

Fairly common in hedgebanks and shady places. Low, creeping and downy. Leaves rounded. Flowers blue-violet or white, sweet-smelling, March to May.

A native of woods and hedgebanks, much cultivated in gardens, and escaped and naturalised far beyond its native range. Its flowers are pleasantly fragrant (though the scent is ephemeral because of its slight anaesthetising effect on smell receptors in the nose).

In the past sweet violet flowers were used quite extensively in cooking for their fragrance and decorative qualities. In the fourteenth century they were beaten up with a ground rice pudding flavoured with ground almonds and cream – and they still make a fine flavouring for rice puddings. The flowers and leaves were both used as ingredients in the elaborate Elizabethan salads known as Grand Salletts or Salmagundies. Much later, after émigrés from the French Revolution had made veal popular in this country, they were used as one of the elaborate floral dressings for joints of that meat. They are best known, though, as crystallised or candied sweets.

Crystallised sweet violets

Pick the flowers, with the stem attached, and dip them first into beaten egg-white and then into a bowl of fine granulated or caster sugar. Use a small paintbrush to coat difficult cavities, as it is important to cover every part with sugar to preserve the flower properly. Let the flowers dry for a few days on greaseproof paper before storing them in an airtight container in the refrigerator.

Garlic Mustard, Jack-by-the-hedge

Alliaria petiolata

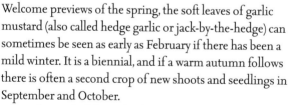

Widespread and plentiful at the edges of woods and on hedgebanks. Height 30–90 cm (1–3 ft). Leaves a fresh, bright green, and slightly toothed. Small, brilliantly white flowers appear April to June.

Welcome previews of the spring, the soft leaves of garlic mustard (also called hedge garlic or jack-by-the-hedge) can sometimes be seen as early as February if there has been a mild winter. It is a biennial, and if a warm autumn follows there is often a second crop of new shoots and seedlings in September and October.

For those who like garlic, but only in moderation, jack-by-the-hedge is ideal as a flavouring. When bruised or chopped the leaves give off just a suspicion of the smell of its unrelated namesake.

Jack-by-the-hedge is a pleasant plant, upright, balanced in colour and classically simple in construction, and only a few leaves should be picked from each specimen. They are useful finely chopped in salads, but best possibly as a sauce for lamb, especially valley lamb, which may well have fed on it in low-lying pastures. In the early spring, chop the leaves with hawthorn buds and a little mint, mix well with vinegar and sugar, and serve with the lamb as you would a mint sauce.

There is also a tradition of using garlic mustard with fish. Gerard recommends this, the seventeenth-century herbalist William Giles reports that it was eaten 'as a sauce to salt fish', and in Wales it accompanied herrings.

• •

Winter-cress

Barbarea vulgaris

Widespread by the sides of roads and streams. Flowers May to July.

It is occasionally sold in markets in the USA, where it is cooked as a green as well as being used as an ingredient of salads. Try picking the young flowers just before they open in May, and stir-frying them as broccoli.

Water-cress

Rorippa nasturtium-aquaticum

Grows abundantly in and beside running water throughout the British Isles. A hairless perennial, creeping or floating, 10–50 cm (4–20 inches). Stem hollow; leaves a rich, silky green. Flowers from June to October in a bunch of small white blossoms.

Now reduced to a steak-house garnish, water-cress was once one of our most respected green vegetables. It was certainly under small-scale cultivation by the middle of the eighteenth century, and quickly became a commercial product as the fast-growing science of nutrition caught a glimpse of its anti-scorbutic properties (which result, as we know now, from an exceptionally high vitamin C content).

Most of the water-cress we eat today is grown commercially, but the cultivated plants are identical in every respect to those that grow wild, sometimes in great green hillocks, on the muddy edges of freshwater streams. The plants to pick are not the young ones, which are rather tasteless, but the older, sturdier specimens, whose darker leaves have a slight burnish to them. These are the tangy ones, which justify the plant's Latin name, *nasi-tortium*, meaning 'nose-twisting'.

Never pick water-cress from stagnant water, or from slow-moving streams that flow through pastureland. It can be a host to one stage in the life-cycle of the liver fluke (*Fasciola hepatica*) which can infest humans as well as sheep and cattle. The larvae are killed by boiling, but it is best to avoid picking specimens that are likely to be infested. Do this by choosing plants in fast-flowing, clean water well out from the riverbank – though this will involve good balance and a sturdy pair of wellingtons.

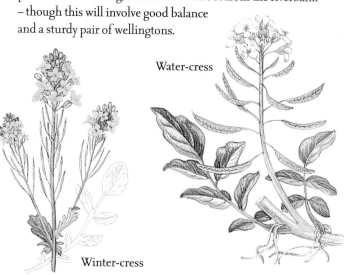

Water-cress

Winter-cress

Do not pull up the plants by the root. Cut off the tops of the shoots and wash them well, wherever they have been growing.

Water-cress makes a good cooked vegetable, especially if spiked with orange and lemon juice and chopped hazelnuts. Simmered with mashed pickled walnuts, it makes a tart sauce for fish.

Water-cress soup

Boil two bunches of water-cress, roughly chopped, in stock made from two large potatoes, 500 ml (1 pint) of water and seasoning. Cook for ten minutes, put through a liquidiser, add a little cream if desired, and serve chilled.

• •

Horse-radish

Armoracia rusticana

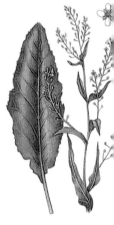

An Asian plant now widely naturalised through much of Europe. Common on waste ground in England and Wales; rare in Scotland and Ireland. Leaves large, slightly toothed, and dock-like, growing straight up from the root stem to a height of about 90 cm (3 ft). Flowers from May to September, a shock of white blossoms on a long spike.

There can scarcely be any other plant of such wide commercial use that is so neglected in the wild. Small jars of horse-radish sauce sell for fancy prices in up-market delicatessens, yet the plant grows untouched and in abundance on waste ground throughout England.

Horse-radish was brought to Britain from the Middle

East in the sixteenth century, specifically as a spice plant. The prefix horse means coarse, as in horse-mint. The rougher the ground, the more horse-radish seems to relish it. It will grow in derelict gardens, on rubbish tips, even amidst abandoned brick piles, regenerating chiefly from pieces of broken root and often quickly developing into large colonies. So you should have no trouble in finding a patch where you can obtain permission to dig up the roots. Remember that the law requires you to obtain the landowner's permission before digging up any wild plant by the root.

There can be no mistaking its crinkly, palm-like leaves, but if you are in any doubt, crush them between your fingers: they should have the characteristic horse-radish smell. A spade – desirable when gathering all roots – is imperative with horse-radish. The plant is a perennial, and carries an extensive and complex root system. You may need to dig quite deep and chop the woody structure to obtain a section for use. The exception is horse-radish growing on light sandy soils, which grows very straight and can often be extracted by a simple pull.

The worst part of preparing horse-radish is the peeling. Most sections are intractably knobbly, and need considerable geometric skill before they can be reduced to a manageable shape. Once they have been, the remains of the brown outer layer should be pared off with a sharp knife. This may be best done under water, as the sharp odour will have started to appear by now. You will be left with some pure white chunks of horse-radish which need to be grated before then can be used. This is best done out of doors, as the fumes put the most blinding onions to shame.

The freshly grated root can be used as it stands, as a garnish for roast beef or smoked fish. But use it fairly quickly, as it loses its potency in a couple of days. Or you can blend it with other ingredients (but under no circumstances vinegar) to make a horse-radish sauce.

Horse-radish sauce (1)

To make an instant sauce, whip up the grated horse-radish with some plain yoghurt or crème fraîche, a little mustard, sugar and seasoning.

Horse-radish sauce (2)

A more substantial and longer-lasting sauce is made by mixing a teaspoon of dry mustard with a tablespoon of cold water, and blending until smooth. Combine with 6 heaped tablespoons of grated horse-radish and salt and pepper. Allow to stand for 15 minutes, then blend into a cupful of white sauce.

. . . .

Hairy Bitter-cress

Cardamine hirsuta

Common and widespread in gardens and waste ground throughout Europe, on paths and walls, also rocks and sand dunes. An annual, 5–25 cm (2–10 inches) high. Leaves compound, cress-like. Flowers white, small, in branched clusters, February to September.

Hairy bitter-cress is one of the earliest edible weeds, with leaves that can be picked most months of the year. The whole plant can be eaten, and it has a pleasantly mild peppery flavour, sweeter than water-cress. It can be used in salads and sandwiches as a substitute for cress, and has an affinity with cream cheese.

Cuckooflower, Lady's-smock

Cardamine pratensis

Common in damp meadows, woods and by the edges of streams. A medium hairless perennial. Flowers April to June.

The leaves are slightly more spicy than those of hairy bitter-cress, and can be used in the same way. The name 'cuckooflower' is shared at a local level with a number of other spring flowers, indicating that their flowering heralds the first cuckoo of the year. The cuckooflower has a traditional use as an ingredient of Easter pudding (see p. 78).

Common Scurvygrass

Cochlearia officinalis

A rather nondescript little plant of coastal cliffs, rocks and salt marshes, also walls and banks. About 10–50 cm (4–20 inches) high, with dark green heart-shaped leaves and small white flowers in loose, domed clusters.

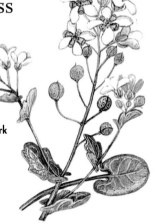

Once famous as the major source of vitamin C on long sea voyages, scurvygrass was taken on board in the form of dried bundles or distilled extracts. But it is an unpleasantly bitter plant, and the taste was often disguised with spices.

But sailors were not the only ones with reason to fear scurvy, and fads for early-morning scurvygrass drinks and scurvygrass sandwiches abounded right up to the middle of the nineteenth century. It was only the ready availability of citrus fruits which finally made the plant obsolete.

Scurvygrass still grows abundantly round cliffs and banks near the sea, and it was probably its convenient proximity that made it the favourite maritime anti-scorbutic.

. . . .

Shepherd's-purse
Capsella bursa-pastoris

Abundant and widespread in waste and cultivated places. A downy, branched annual, 5–60 cm (2–24 inches). Leaves spear-shaped and deeply lobed, in a neat basal rosette. Flowers small with white petals and pink calyx. Fruit is small, heart-shaped pods.

Shepherd's-purse is one of the first wild plants to flower, and will sometimes flower all through mild winters. It is slightly peppery in taste, and is popular in China, where it is stir-fried, like cabbage and Chinese leaf.

Field Penny-cress

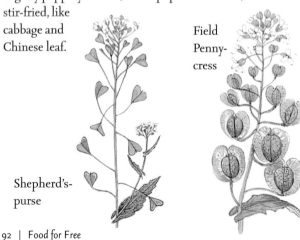

Shepherd's-purse

Field Penny-cress
Thlaspi arvense

Quite common in arable and waste places. Flowers May to November.

As is the case with all the wild members of the cabbage family, field penny-cress can be used in the same way as chickweed, either in salads or as cooked greens.

• •

Dittander
Lepidium latifolium

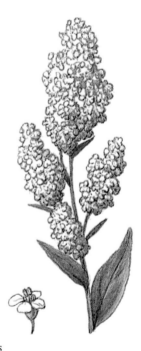

A robust perennial of salt marshes, sand dunes and other places near salt water. Up to 1 m (3 ft) high. Lower leaves long, up to 30 cm (1 ft). Flowers in a white cluster, July to September.

Dittander has a hot, pungent root, and was gathered from the wild and occasionally grown in gardens as a condiment before horse-radish and pepper became popular. It is a perennial and has an obstinate and aggressive root system like horse-radish, yet is now uncommon in the wild. Only beside a few estuaries on the south and east coasts can the tall, elegant leaves and robust flower spires still be found.

Wild Cabbage

Brassica oleracea

A hairless perennial of sea cliffs and rocks, on dry stony soils, up to 1.5 m (5 ft) high. Leaves greyish, lower ones large and lobed, upper ones unlobed and partly clasping the stem. Flowers yellow, in long clusters, May to September.

This scarce plant of the sea cliffs in parts of Wales and southern England is a variety of the same species as our cultivated cabbages, but it is uncertain whether it is the ancestor of those cultivated varieties, or whether the wild species originated from cultivated forms in ancient settlements. Today the plant is rare in its natural habitat. Yet escaped garden *Brassicas* sometimes revert to this form if they are allowed to go to seed. You can tell them easily from the mustards and other related plants by their thick, greyish, fleshy leaves. They are bitter raw, but after long simmering are acceptable to eat.

Black Mustard

Brassica nigra

Quite common as an escape from cultivation on waysides and waste places. Tall, greyish-green annual, up to 1 m (3 ft) high. Leaves stalked, lower ones lobed and bristly. Flowers yellow, June to August. Fruit in the form of seed-pods pressed against the stem.

Use the young leaves of black mustard as a tangy addition to spring salads and cooked greens. The seeds begin to ripen in August to September, and have long been used in cooking. Collecting them can be a painstaking business, and you are unlikely to gather more than a pinch, but try pressing some into the cheese on the top of a Welsh rarebit before cooking. Slightly more seeds will be enough to make a chutney.

Lemon and mustard-seed chutney

4 onions
5 lemons
Salt
25 g (1 oz) black mustard seed
1 teaspoon allspice
500 g (1 lb) sugar
100 g (4 oz) raisins
500 ml (1 pint) cider vinegar

1 Thinly slice the onions and lemons, sprinkle with salt and leave for 12 hours.
2 Add the mustard seeds, allspice, sugar, raisins and vinegar.
3 Bring to the boil and simmer for 1 hour.
4 Transfer to jars and seal when cool.

• •

White Mustard

Sinapis alba

A common weed in arable land, and an escape from cultivation, especially on chalky soils. Flowers May to October. This is the mustard of 'mustard and cress'.

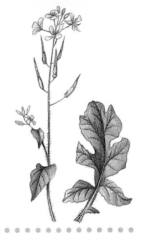

Under cultivation the plants are picked when they are only a few centimetres high. In the wild they need to be picked rather later for certain identification, by which time they tend to be slightly bitter. Use as chickweed in spring salads or in cooked greens.

Sea-kale

Crambe maritima

Widespread but extremely local on sand and shingle near the sea. A cabbage-like plant, growing in large clumps with huge fleshy grey-green leaves. The flowers are white and four-petalled, and grow in a broad cluster, June to August.

Up to the nineteenth century sea-kale was a relatively common plant around the coasts, and there is little doubt that the use of the plant dates back centuries before it was taken into cultivation. In many areas on the south coast villagers would watch for the shoots to appear, pile sand and shingle round them to blanch out the bitterness and cut them in the summer to take to the markets in the nearest big town. But in 1799 the botanist William Curtis wrote a pamphlet called *Directions for the culture of the Crambe Maritima or Sea kale, for the use of the Table*. As a result the vegetable was taken up by Covent Garden, and demand for the naturally growing shoots increased greatly. This intensive collection was to have the effect of substantially reducing the population of wild sea-kale.

Now the vegetable is out of fashion, but the wild plant shows no sign of regaining its former status. So be sparing if you do pick it, and do not take more than two or three stems from each plant. Use young shoots or the lower parts of the leaf stalks, particularly any that you can find which have been growing under the ground. They sometimes push their way through up to a metre (3 ft) of shingle, and when harvesting you will need a sharp knife to cut through the thick stems.

To cook the sea-kale, cut the stems into manageable lengths and boil in salted water until tender (about 20 minutes). Then serve and eat with melted butter, like asparagus. Alternatively, use lemon juice or sauce hollandaise. The very young shoots and leaves can also be eaten raw as a salad.

Sea-kale and pasta

2 handfuls of mixed stems, leaf-shoots and small flower-heads of sea-kale
500 g (1 lb) penne pasta
Chopped anchovies
2 tablespoons olive oil
Butter
Lemon juice

1 Chop the sea-kale into 5 cm (2 inch) lengths and cook in boiling water for about 10 minutes.
2 Add the penne to salted boiling water and simmer until just cooked (8–10 minutes).
3 Drain the pasta, add the cooked sea-kale, a few chopped anchovies, the olive oil, a knob of butter and a squeeze of lemon. Stir and heat for a further 3 minutes, then serve.

Crowberry

Empetrum nigrum

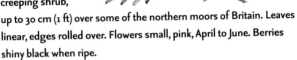

A small,
creeping shrub,
up to 30 cm (1 ft) over some of the northern moors of Britain. Leaves linear, edges rolled over. Flowers small, pink, April to June. Berries shiny black when ripe.

The fruits are used in arctic regions and probably have some value as a source of vitamin C. Although it is difficult to gather the fruit in any quantity some experimenters have enjoyed jelly made from it.

Heather

Calluna vulgaris

Widespread and abundant on heaths, moors, and dry, open woods on acid soils. An evergreen shrub up to 1 m (3 ft) high, with numerous tiny leaves in opposite rows. The flowers are purple and bell-shaped and carried in spikes, August to September.

Heather is the dominant plant over much of western Europe's upland moors and sandy wastes. In full flower – purple billows as far as the eye can see – a heather moor is a glorious sight. But it is also a deceptive one, for heather is a sign of a depleted soil and a harsh climate. Heather is a tenacious plant and completely carpets huge areas of moorland. Trample on it and you will make no impression on its wiry stems. Even extensive burning only sets it back temporarily, and within a couple of years new shoots spring up beside the blackened branches of the old.

Heather has an abundant range of economic uses. It provides food for sheep and grouse, material for fuel, thatching, basketwork and brooms, and an orange dye. Its flowers are rich in nectar, and beekeepers often transport their hives many miles to a stretch of moorland when the heather is in bloom. The dried flower-heads make a good tea, and Robert Burns is supposed to have drunk a 'moorland tea' based on heather tops mixed with the dried leaves of bilberry, blackberry, speedwell, thyme and wild strawberry.

Heather ale has a long history in Scotland, dating back to the Neolithic period. The tradition was revived commercially in the late twentieth century, and heather ale is now available under the Gaelic name of Fraoch. It is wonderfully fragrant, with scents of heather and honey.

Bilberry
Vaccinium myrtillus

Widespread throughout the British Isles, except the south and east of England, and locally abundant on heaths and moors. An erect shrub, growing 20–50 cm (8–20 inches) high, with hairless twigs and oval, slightly toothed, bright green leaves. Flowers solitary, drooping, greenish-pink globes. Fruits small, round and blue-black, covered with bloom, July to September

Also known as whortleberries or whinberries, and in Scotland as blaeberries, bilberries transport you more thoroughly into the role of the hunter-gatherer than perhaps any other wild food. The fruit is virtually unknown in cultivation – the blueberries bought from greengrocers and supermarkets are a larger and less flavoursome American species.

The bilberry is an intriguingly juicy and versatile fruit, and would doubtless be more popular commercially if picking it were not such a laborious business. The shrub grows low, often largely concealed by dense heather, and the berries form in nothing like the concentrations of, say, blackberries. So even on the moors where the bush grows in abundance, gathering any quantity can involve the thorough searching of a fair-sized patch of land. On parts of mainland Europe, bilberry gathering has been partially mechanised with the help of a large combing device known as a *peigne*, though this not only damages the more fragile shoots and strips many of the leaves along with the berries but also takes away much of the fun of hunting for the berries – the discovery of clusters of fruit under the leaves, and one's fingers (and mouth) turning blue.

In Britain the wild fruit is still picked commercially on a small scale, particularly in the Welsh border country, where the berries are sold in markets. Bilberries can be used to make jams, jellies, stews and cheesecakes. They can be frozen, or left to stand in the sun for a week or so, by which time they will have dried sufficiently to keep over the winter.

Some of the most interesting bilberry recipes come from Yorkshire, where the pies are known as 'mucky-mouth pies' because of the colour they give to tongues and lips. Another Yorkshire touch with bilberries is to add a few sprigs of mint to the stewed fruit and jams. The two flavours complement each other perfectly.

Bilberry pudding

A classic recipe which sets the berries in a kind of Yorkshire pudding.

100 g (4 oz) flour
1 egg
1 large cup of milk
2 tablespoons brown sugar
200 g (8 oz) bilberries

1 Make a thinnish batter by beating the egg with the flour and then slowly adding the milk.
2 Stir in the sugar and the bilberries and pour into a greased tin.
3 Bake in a medium oven for 30 minutes.

Cranberry

Vaccinium oxycoccos

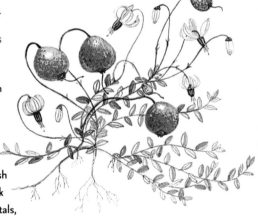

A creeping, evergreen shrub of bogs and marshy heaths, up to 50 cm (20 inches) high. Leaves dark green, pointed, whitish beneath. Flowers pink with down-turned petals, June to August. Berries small, round, mottled red.

Cranberries were once more common in Britain. But the draining of much of our marsh and upland bog has robbed the plant of its natural wet habitats, and it is now largely confined to the north of England and Wales.

The berry of the wild plant is inedible raw, and you are unlikely to find enough for cooking. But it can be made into sauce like the larger American species. In fact, its origins, name and traditional uses are solidly British, and the fruit is mentioned (as 'fenberry') in a herbal published in 1578. Like so much else, cranberry recipes were preserved by British settlers in America, and only later brought back into use here.

Cowberry
Vaccinium vitis-idaea

A small evergreen shrub of moorland bogs, 40 cm (16 inches) high. Leaves leathery, oval, untoothed. Flowers pink or white, in clusters, May to July. Berries red, spherical.

Also known as lingonberry, this little shrub is a close relative of the cranberry, and one of its names is in fact mountain cranberry. It grows on some moors in the northern parts of the British Isles, and more widely in northern Europe. They are popular in Sweden, where they are known as 'the red gold of the forests'. Like cranberries, the berries are sharp and scarcely edible when raw, and are usually made into jam or jelly (though they need some apple added for the pectin).

Cowslip
Primula veris

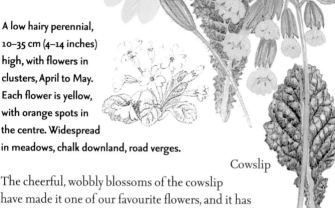

Primrose

A low hairy perennial, 10–35 cm (4–14 inches) high, with flowers in clusters, April to May. Each flower is yellow, with orange spots in the centre. Widespread in meadows, chalk downland, road verges.

Cowslip

The cheerful, wobbly blossoms of the cowslip have made it one of our favourite flowers, and it has probably suffered more from overpicking than any other of our once-common meadow flowers. Yet its name hardly suggests such popularity. It is a euphemism for 'cowslop', no doubt an indication of the plant's liking for mucky fields.

It was once widely used in kitchens, making one of the very best country wines, and a curious 'vinegar' which was drunk with soda water rather than being used as a condiment. (To show the devastation some of these recipes must have wreaked on flower populations, this particular recipe required two pints of cowslip blossoms to make a pint and a half of vinegar.)

The picking of wild flowers is strongly discouraged these days because of declining populations. If you like the sound of any of the recipes, grow the plants in your garden – or even in a window box – and pick the flowers there. Many species, such as cowslip and primrose, are commercially available as seed.

Primrose

Primula vulgaris

A low hairy perennial, 10–25 cm (4–10 inches) high, with crinkly leaves and pale yellow flowers, March to May. Widespread throughout Europe, in woodland and on hedgebanks, railway embankments and cliffs.

The symbol of spring, with its pure, pale, delicately fragrant yellow flowers, the primrose can grow abundantly on chalk banks, shady woods, even on cliffs, but it is often greatly reduced near towns and cities because of uprooting. Primrose blossoms have mostly been used in similar ways to cowslips and violets – strewn on salads and on roast meats, candied, or made into wine – but they are not common enough in most places today to justify picking from the wild.

Red Currant

Ribes rubrum

Widespread but local in woods and hedgerows, especially by streams and fens. An erect shrub, up to 1.5 m (5 ft) high, with toothed leaves broken into 3 or 5 lobes, not aromatic. Flowers small, green and drooping, April and May. Fruits from July, round and shiny red, with a slightly translucent skin.

Some red currant bushes are blatant escapes from nearby gardens. But the plant is an authentic native, and truly wild specimens are not uncommon in old woodland, by stream banks and in rough fens.

The fruits appear from July, and are often much less red than their cultivated cousins. Avoid confusion with the cloying fruit of guelder-rose (Viburnum opulus). This is also a shrub of woods and riversides, but its berries lack a 'tail' and look heavy and waxy beside the almost translucent skins of the red currant.

Red currants make a good jelly, provided the rather obtrusive pips are strained out. But given that you will probably only find a few, they may be best eaten as a bracing field-snack, in what the fruit gourmet Edward Bunyard described as 'ambulant consumption'.

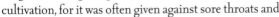

Black Currant

Ribes nigrum

Grows wild in damp woodland across the whole of Europe. An erect shrub, up to 1.5 m (5 ft) high, with lobed leaves which issue a heavy and characteristic smell when crushed. Flowers drooping, April and May. Dangling clusters of opaque black berries appear in June, ripening in July.

The soothing properties of black currant juice were probably known long before the plant passed into cultivation, for it was often given against sore throats and 'the quinsy'. It is a rather uncommon plant in the wild, and can readily be told from red currant by its larger, heavily aromatic leaves. A few of these, dried, can transform a pot of Indian tea.

The currants can also be dried, and in this form they were one of the bases of pemmican, an Amerindian dish taken up by polar explorers. The currants were pounded together with dried meat, and the mixture bound together and coated with fat or tallow. The result was a food containing almost all the ingredients necessary for a balanced diet, which would keep well even on long journeys.

Black currant jam

Remove the stalks from 2 kg (4 lb) of black currants, and put in a large pan with 500 ml (1 pint) of water. Bring to the boil and simmer until the fruit is tender (about 30 minutes), then add 2 kg (4 lb) of sugar and make sure it has dissolved completely before bringing it back to the boil. Boil for about 15 minutes, until the setting point is reached, then remove from the heat and pot in the usual way.

Gooseberry
Ribes uva-crispa

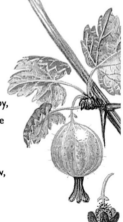

Widespread but scattered in woods and hedgerows across most of Europe. A stubby, many-branched shrub, rarely growing more than 120 cm (4 ft) high, with 3- or 4-lobed, blunt-toothed leaves, and drooping, red-tinged, green flowers. Fruit greenish yellow, egg-shaped and usually hairy, from July.

Although some gooseberries found in the wild are naturalised from bird-sown garden varieties, the species is almost certainly native. The history of the gooseberry's domestication, from lowly hedgerow berry to luscious dessert fruit, is one of the most extraordinary stories of vernacular plant breeding. Cultivated gooseberries were unknown until late in the sixteenth century, yet by the end of the nineteenth there were as many as 2,000 named varieties. This was due almost entirely to the ingenuity of amateur growers, especially in the industrial Midlands, who were spurred on in their breeding programmes by annual competitions (still held in a few villages).

You will find wild gooseberries from early July onwards, and on some bushes (with the help of a pair of gloves, because of the spines) you may be able to pick a fair quantity, though they are irregular fruiters. Depending on their ripeness and sweetness they can be used in any of the recipes which normally employ the cultivated fruit. The ripe berries make gooseberry pie or gooseberry fool, the under-ripe ones gooseberry jelly (see the recipe for elderflower and gooseberry preserve on p. 56).

Oldbury tarts, from Oldbury-on-Severn, were traditionally made with wild gooseberries and sold at the Whitsuntide fairs (though the berries can hardly have been ripe at this time, and preserved fruit must have been used). The tarts were actually small pies, tea-cup sized, filled with gooseberries and demerara sugar.

Gooseberry and fennel sauce

This requires only a small quantity of berries, and goes well with mackerel. Stew a handful of fruit in a little cider, pulp through a sieve, then mix with chopped fennel (p. 139). Add mustard and honey to taste.

Gooseberry fool

1 cup wild gooseberries
½ cup double cream
2 glasses white wine
1 tablespoon honey
Wild rose petals to garnish

1 Top and tail the gooseberries. Stew in the white wine and honey, and reduce until the mixture is the consistency of jam.
2 Whip the cream until stiff.
3 When the gooseberry mixture is cool, fold in the whipped cream and decorate with rose petals.

Opposite-leaved Golden-saxifrage
Chrysosplenium oppositifolium

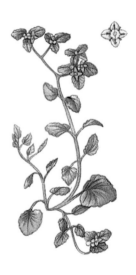

A low, creeping plant with a preference for the banks of springs and wet, shady mountainsides.

In the Vosges mountains the leaves of this golden-saxifrage are eaten under the name *cresson de roches*. It can be used as a green vegetable, but it is not common enough to justify picking, except where plentiful.

Meadowsweet

Filipendula ulmaria

Widespread and often abundant throughout the British Isles, by fresh water, in fens and marshy places and damp woods. A hairy perennial, 60–120 cm (2–4 ft) high. Leaves toothed, dark green above, silvery grey below. Foamy clusters of cream-coloured flowers on stiff, reddish-tinged stems, June to October.

One of the most summery of all our wild plants. In July the frothy flower-heads of meadowsweet can transform a riverside meadow. The scent of the fresh flowers is warm and heady, that of the crushed leaves more clinically sharp. When dried, both parts of the plant smell of new-mown hay. It was these dried leaves that were used to give an especially aromatic bouquet to port, claret and mead, and it is to this function that the name 'meadwort' probably refers, rather than to its preference for growing in meadows. The leaves can be used for flavouring almost any sort of drink, and can double for woodruff (p. 162) if that plant is unobtainable.

Raspberry

Rubus idaeus

Widespread throughout the British Isles, and quite frequent in hedgerows, rocky woods, and heaths. A slender shrub, with usually unbranched arching stems growing up to 2 m (6 ft) high, and only very slightly spiny. Leaves toothed and oval, and often whitish below. Flowers small and white in drooping clusters. Fruit a rich red berry, formed by a number of drupelets, July to September.

Although many raspberry plants growing in the wild are bird-seeded from cultivated stock, the fruit is as authentic a British native as its close relative the blackberry. It is not difficult to see why, of the two, it was the raspberry that was taken into gardens. It grows more tidily and with greater restraint than the spiny, aggressive bramble. And this of course means that it has been less prolific in the wild – another good reason for nurturing the plant in the non-competitive security of the garden.

The raspberry is usually the first soft fruit to ripen, occasionally as early as the last weeks of June. If you have difficulty distinguishing young raspberries from unripe blackberries, look at the stems on which they are growing. The raspberry has woody, cane-like stems, comparatively smooth except for a few weak prickles; the blackberry has much coarser stems armed with a great number of strong prickles. The berries themselves are quite different in texture, even when they are similarly coloured. Raspberries have a matt, spongy surface, whilst blackberries are covered with a shiny, taut skin. And when fully ripe the raspberry comes away easily from its pithy core.

Raspberries are such a rich and substantial fruit that it would be a waste to make jelly from them. But simmered in their own juice for about a quarter of an hour, and then boiled to setting point with an equal weight of sugar, they make a fine jam. If you only find a handful of wild berries, use them for stuffing game birds, or to make the famous summer pudding.

Raspberry vinegar, which can be made by soaking 450 g (1 lb) of fruit in 500 ml (1 pint) of white wine vinegar for two or three days, is an important ingredient of *nouvelle cuisine*. But it has an ancient pedigree as a sauce for fruit dishes and a base for summer drinks, and as a popular domestic remedy for 'tickly' throats.

Summer pudding

8–10 slices of bread (brown or white), Milk
600 g (1½ lb) summer fruits, such as raspberries, red and black currants, Sugar to taste

1 Cut some fairly thin slices of bread and remove the crusts. Moisten with milk, and line the sides and bottom of a deep pudding basin with them. Make sure that the slices overlap well, so that they will hold together when turned out.

2 Fill the basin with the fruit mixture, which should have been cooked for about 10 minutes and sweetened with sugar to taste.

3 Cover the top with more slices of moistened bread, and then with greaseproof paper. Put a weight on top of the paper and leave the pudding to stand in the refrigerator overnight.

4 Turn out and serve with crème fraîche or ice-cream.

Blackberry, Bramble

Rubus fruticosus

Widespread and abundant in woods, hedges, waste places and heaths. A prickly shrub, usually growing in straggly, tangled clumps. The leaves are also prickly and toothed, and turn reddish-purple in

the autumn. The flowers have 5 white or pinkish petals. The fruit is made up of a number of drupelets, and turns from green to red to a deep purple-black. It can be picked from August to October.

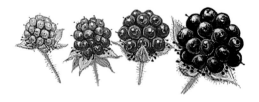

There is little need to write at length about this juicy purple berry, which has been known, loved and picked across the world for generations. Its seeds have even been found in the stomach of a Neolithic man dug up from the Essex clay. Blackberries have a special role in the relationship between townspeople and the countryside. It is not just that they are delicious, and easy to find. Blackberrying carries with it a little of the urban dweller's myth of country life: abundance, harvest, a sense of season, and just enough discomfort to quicken the senses. Maybe it is the scuffing and the scratches that are the real attraction of blackberrying, the proof of satisfying toil against unruly nature.

Everyone has their favourite picking habits and recipes, and these are better guides than anything a book can say. So I will confine myself here to a few of the lesser known facts.

Blackberry bushes spread in a curious way. Each cane begins by growing erectly, but then curves downwards until its tip touches the ground. Here the shoot takes root, and a clump of new canes soon forms. The berries themselves grow in large clusters at the end of the older shoots, which die after two or three years' cropping. The lowest berry – right at the tip of the stalk – is the first to ripen, and is the sweetest and fattest of all. Eat it raw. A few weeks later, the other berries near the end ripen; these are less juicy, but are still good for jam and pies. The small berries farther up the stalk often do not ripen until October. They are hard and slightly bitter and are only really useful if cooked with some other fruit.

Even more variety is found from bush to bush. There are reckoned to be at least 400 microspecies in Britain, all differing slightly in flavour, sweetness, fruiting time, nutritional content and size. Blackberries can occur with the savours of grape, plum and even apple. Some varieties have more dietary fibre, weight for weight, than wholemeal bread. If any wild variety does take your fancy, try growing a cutting in the garden. It should bear fruit after a couple of years.

There are any number of recipes which make use of blackberries. They can be made into pies, fruit fools and salads, jellies (they need a little extra pectin), and jams. A good way of serving them fresh is to leave them to steep overnight in red wine.

The most delicious blackberry product I know is a junket made from nothing other than blackberry juice. Remove the juice from the very ripest berries with the help of a juice extractor, or by pressing them through several layers of muslin. Then simply allow the thick, dark juice to stand undisturbed in a warm room. Do not stir or cool the juice, or add anything to it. In a few hours it will have set to the consistency of a light junket, and can be eaten with cream and sweet biscuits.

Autumn pudding

Make as for summer pudding (see p. 111), but replace the bright red fruits with dark ones – blackberries especially, and also a few stoned sloes and damsons, elderberries, and chopped crab apples. Cook for about ten minutes and stir in dark honey or sugar to taste. Transfer the pulp to a deep pudding basin lined with slices of wholemeal bread, and pack in more bread until the pulp is covered. Put a weight on top and leave in the refrigerator overnight.

Dewberry

Rubus caesius

**Widespread and frequent in bushy and
grassy places, especially in eastern England.
Hairy, sprawling perennial, up to 40 cm (16 inches)
high, with weak prickles.**

The dewberry carries smaller fruits than the blackberry.
They have fewer segments and are covered with a fine
bloom. They are also so juicy that they can be difficult to
pick without bursting. Take advantage of this juiciness and
pick them as a kind of ready-made cocktail cherry. Snip a
few of the best berries off with secateurs, together with
about 8 cm (3 inches) of stalk. Serve them with their 'sticks'
intact, ready for dipping in bowls of sugar and cream.

Cloudberry

Rubus chamaemorus

**This little shrub, which grows not much more than
15 cm (6 inches) high, is a relative of the blackberry.
It grows in patches on damp peatland soils.
Fruit red at first, orange when ripe.**

Sadly, the cloudberry has always been a shy fruiter in this
country (unlike Scandinavia, for instance, where it is highly
prized). It is a subalpine and arctic species, confined to bogs
and moors in Scotland and the north of England and Wales.

In the Berwyn mountains in north Wales, an unusual
tradition commemorated this scarcity, and persisted up to

the end of the nineteenth century. Shepherds from Llanrhaiadr believed that a quart of cloudberries was the wage that St Dogfan was due for his spiritual ministry, and anyone who could bring such a quantity to the parson on St Dogfan's Day had his tithes (taxes) remitted for the year.

Cloudberries have been used in northern areas of Britain for puddings or jams, and could be included in any dish that is conventionally made from blackberries or raspberries.

Silverweed

Potentilla anserina

An abundant flower of damp grassy and waste places. A hairy, creeping perennial, 10–30 cm (4–12 inches) high. Leaves in a basal rosette, coarsely toothed. Flowers yellow, five-petalled, May to September.

The undersides of the leaves are flashed with a pale matt grey, making the plant look withered before its time. The upper surface is a silky, liquid green. The leaves were once used by foot soldiers as an apparently cooling lining for their boots. The whole plant has a history of medicinal and culinary use going back to the ancient Greeks.

The roots were cultivated as a crop from late prehistoric times. In upland areas of Britain they were eaten right up until the introduction of the potato – and later, in times of famine, though they are a meagre and not very flavoursome root. The seventeenth-century botanist John Ray likened their taste to parsnip. The roots were boiled, baked, or even eaten raw; they were also dried and ground into flour for bread and gruel.

Silverweed is worth bringing into your garden for its ambivalent leaves and yellow, utilitarian flowers. If you do, some of those old famine recipes for the roots are worth reviving.

- -

Wild Strawberry

Fragaria vesca

Widespread and frequent on grassy banks, heaths, open woods throughout Europe. A low, creeping plant with hairy runners and stems 5–30 cm (2–12 inches). The leaves are in groups of three, toothed, shiny green above and silky grey beneath. The fruits are small drooping red berries with the seeds protruding, late June to September.

In some parts of the country wild strawberries are abundant, and carpet wide patches of dry and heathy ground. But normally you will need to search carefully for them, looking for the trefoil leaves in the bracken edges and rough grass. The drooping berries can be even more elusive, and are often completely hidden by the leaves. Always look under the leaves as well as on top of the plant when picking wild strawberries.

Wild strawberries prefer chalky soils, and the best fruits are those eaten straight from plants growing on bare limestone. They will have been warmed up by the sun reflected from the rock, and their fragrance can be savoured to the full.

What the wild strawberry lacks in size it more than makes up for in flavour.

The ripe fruits are wonderfully concentrated beads of sweetness, which our ancestors appreciated in much the same way as we do. The most useful recipes are those which make the best of small quantities of berries. Try a wineglassful topped with champagne. Add a few to a fresh fruit salad – or a green salad, for that matter. Or make use of their winey aroma by turning them into a sauce for other fruit, especially raspberries or peaches. Simply purée them with a little wine, pepper and sugar.

Herb-bennet, Wood Avens

Geum urbanum

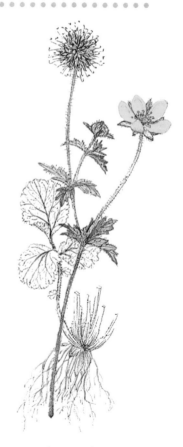

An undistinguished plant, yet it is pleasant in late summer to find its small five-petalled yellow flowers on an otherwise dark woodland floor.

The clove-like odour of the roots of herb-bennet was once reputed to repel moths; yet it clearly attracted human beings, for it was widely grown as a pot-herb in the sixteenth century. As well as its many medicinal uses (against 'the stings of venomous beasts') it was also added to broths and soups.

Salad Burnet

Sanguisorba minor

**Quite common in grassy places on chalk.
A hairless perennial, 20–90 cm (8–36 inches),
with four to twelve pairs of oval, toothed leaves.
Flowers green, reddish or purplish, May to August.**

When crushed, the leaves of the salad burnet
smell slightly of cucumber. They have long been
used as an ingredient of salads, in spite of their diminutive
size and slight bitterness, and as a garnish for summer drinks.

    Sir Francis Bacon recommended that salad burnet
should be planted in herb gardens with wild thyme and
water mint, 'to perfume the air most delightfully, being
trodden on and crushed'. A recipe reputedly enjoyed by
Napoleon whilst he was in exile on St Helena was a salad of
cooked haricot beans, dressed with a generous mixture of
olive oil and green herbs – salad burnet (*pimprenelles* in
French), tarragon, chives, parsley and chervil.

Parsley-piert

Aphanes arvensis

**Widespread and common on arable and dry ground.
Very low, hairy, pale green annual with lobed, toothed
leaves. Flowers tiny, green, in clusters, April to October.**

The curious name of this plant probably derives
from *perce-pierre*, a plant which breaks
through stony ground. So, by sympathetic magic,

it came to be used medicinally as a specific against kidney stones. Yet it was Culpeper of all people, herbal wizard extraordinary, who first recommended it as an honest domestic pickle. Best as a small-scale addition to salads.

- -

Wild Rose, Dog-rose

Rosa canina

Widespread and common in hedges, scrubland, waste places, but less frequent in Scotland. A thorny plant with arching stems up to 3 m (10 ft) high, with hooked prickles, toothed leaves, and large, white to pink, five-petalled flowers, June and July. The fruit (rosehip) is an orange-red, oblong berry, sometimes as much as 2.5 cm (1 inch) long, and is on the bushes between late August and November.

The wild rose has a simpler and less showy blossom than the garden rose and scarcely droops before it sheds its petals. This is the stage when wild roses should be gathered. Never pick or damage the young flowers. Towards the end of July look for those that have already lost one or two petals, and then gently remove the others into your basket.

Wild roses have a more delicate scent than the garden varieties, but still some of that fleshy, perfumed texture. So if you have only a small quantity, use them neat in salads. Frances Perry once listed ten other uses for the petals: rose wine, rose in brandy, rose vinegar, rhubarb and rose-petal jam, rose honey, rose and coconut candies, Turkish delight, rose drops, crystallised rose petals, and rose-petal jelly. The list could be extended indefinitely, because the basis of the use of rose-petals, here as elsewhere, is simply as a fragrant improver of well-established dishes.

Rose-petal jam

Extensively eaten in the Middle Fast, especially with yoghurt; this recipe is from Turkey. You will only need to prepare a small potful, as it is exceedingly sweet. And only supplement your wild petals with those from garden roses if it is absolutely necessary to make up the quantity: the thick, fleshy petals of the garden damasks are very difficult to reduce to jelly.

2 cups wild rose petals (crammed down fairly tightly)
2 cups sugar, 1 cup water
1 tablespoon lemon juice
1 tablespoon orange juice

1 Dissolve the sugar in the water, and add the lemon juice and orange juice.
2 Make sure that the rose petals are free of insects, and discard any withered ones.
3 Stir the petals into the liquid and put the pan over a very low heat. Stir continuously for about 30 minutes, or until all the petals have 'melted'.
4 Cool a little, pour into a small glass jar and cover.

Rosehips

The fruit of the wild rose, the hip, is the star of one of the great success stories of wild food use. It is the only completely wild fruit to have supported a national commercial enterprise – the production of rosehip syrup.

The austerity of the Second World War, when supplies of citrus fruits were virtually cut off, forced the British government to exploit the potential of rosehips as a source of vitamin C. But the fruit had been used as a food for centuries before that. When cultivated fruit was scarce in the

Middle Ages, rosehips were used as a dessert. A recipe from 1730 explains how this hard, unlikely berry was transformed into a filling for tarts. The hips were first split in half, and the pith and seeds thoroughly cleaned out. Then the skins were put to stand in an earthenware pot until they were soft enough to rub through a sieve. (Notice that this was done without the use of any heat or liquid.) The resulting purée was mixed with its own weight of sugar, warmed until the sugar melted, and then potted.

In 1941 the Ministry of Health put forward a scheme for collection of rosehips, which had been found to contain twenty times the amount of vitamin C in oranges, and in that year 120 tons were gathered by voluntary collectors. The next year the scheme was transferred to the Vegetable Drugs Committee of the Ministry of Supply and 344 tons were gathered. By 1943 the redoubtable County Herb Committees were brought in to organise the collection, and for the next three years the harvest averaged 450 tons. The resulting syrup was sold through ordinary retailers at a controlled price of 1s 9d a six-ounce (170 ml) bottle. Mothers and children were able to obtain it in larger quantities, and at reduced prices, from Welfare Clinics. Rosehip syrup stayed in the shops through the 1960s and 1970s, but it is now commercially available only from specialist suppliers.

Rosehip syrup is really the beginning of all useful rosehip recipes, and making it is the simplest way of filtering out the prickly seed, which can be a dangerous internal irritant. Here, as a nostalgic but highly functional guide, are the meticulous directions given by the Ministry of Food during the Second World War for 900 g (2 lb) of hips. The resulting syrup can be used as a flavouring for milk puddings, ice-cream or almost any sweet, or diluted as a drink.

Rosehip syrup

Have ready 3 pints [1.5 litres] of boiling water, mince
the hips in a coarse mincer, drop immediately into
the boiling water or if possible mince the hips directly
into the boiling water and again bring to the boil.
Stop heating and place aside for 15 minutes. Pour
into a flannel or linen crash jelly bag and allow to drip
until the bulk of the liquid has come through. Return
the residue to the saucepan, add 1½ pints [750 ml] of
boiling water, stir and allow to stand for 10 minutes.
Pour back into the jelly bag and allow to drip. To make
sure all the sharp hairs are removed put back the first
half cupful of liquid and allow to drip through again.
Put the mixed juice into a clean saucepan and boil
down until the juice measures about 1½ pints
[750 ml], then add 1½ lbs [900 g] of sugar and boil for
a further 5 minutes. Pour into hot sterile bottles and
seal at once. If corks are used these should have been
boiled for ½ hour just previously and after insertion
coated with melted paraffin wax. It is advisable to use
small bottles as the syrup will not keep for more than
a week or two once the bottle is opened. Store in a
dark cupboard.

Hedgerow Harvest, Ministry of Food, 1943

· ·

Bitter-vetch

Lathyrus linifolius

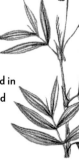

A short, erect, hairless perennial with
winged stems, up to 40 cm (16 inches), found in
damp grassland and open woods. Purple-red
flowers, fading to blue, April to July.

An edible tuber from the pea family, bitter-vetch is one of the commoner species, and sometimes grows in abundance in heathy areas. It has been recognised as a vegetable since at least the Middle Ages. In later times the roots were used as a subsistence crop in the Scottish islands, either raw or dried. They have also been used for flavouring whisky.

Restharrow

Ononis repens

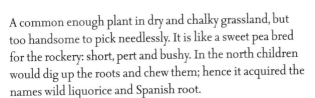

Hairy, sticky, spreading perennial, 10–70 cm (4–28 inches), found in lime-rich soil in grassland, shingle, sand dunes. Loose clusters of pink-purple flowers, June to September.

A common enough plant in dry and chalky grassland, but too handsome to pick needlessly. It is like a sweet pea bred for the rockery: short, pert and bushy. In the north children would dig up the roots and chew them; hence it acquired the names wild liquorice and Spanish root.

Rosebay Willowherb

Chamerion angustifolium

Widespread and abundant in woodland clearings and on waste ground, especially where there has been fire. Pink flowers in dramatic spikes up to 1.5 m (5 ft) high, June to September.

The young shoots have been eaten like asparagus in parts of America and northern Europe, though they are very bitter.

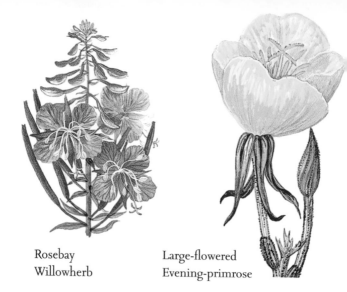

Rosebay
Willowherb

Large-flowered
Evening-primrose

Large-flowered
Evening-primrose
Oenothera glazioviana

A tall, downy flower, up to 1.8 m (6 ft), with a fine poppy-like yellow
blossom.

Introduced from America into Britain in the early
seventeenth century, and soon taken into gardens for its
roots, which were eaten boiled. In Germany the young
shoots were also eaten.

. . . .

Dwarf Cornel

Cornus suecica

A short, creeping perennial, up to 20 cm (8 inches), found on upland
moors. Purplish flowers appear in June to August. The fruits are red.

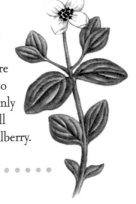

The one aperitif in this book. The small scarlet berries used to be munched by the Highlanders to stimulate their appetites.

Dwarf cornel is rare, and there are more agreeable ways to perk up your appetite, so this rare plant should be left unpicked. Only in a few areas in the Highlands does it still thrive under the shelter of heather and bilberry.

- -

Dog's Mercury
Mercurialis perennis
☠ POISONOUS

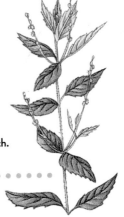

A low, unbranched, downy perennial, often growing in large colonies in woods, and under ancient hedgebanks. Tassels of small, yellowish-green flowers in early spring. Dog's Mercury contains an intensely irritant poison which can damage the liver and kidneys as well as the stomach.

- -

Spurge
Euphorbia species
☠ POISONOUS

Modest-looking plants commonly regarded as weeds. Yellowish-green flowers from April to September, depending on the species.

The majority of our native spurges are poisonous. They exude a milky juice which can produce intense irritation of the lips and mouth, and act as a drastic purgative if swallowed. Sun spurge, *Euphorbia helioscopia*, dwarf spurge, *Euphorbia exigua*, and petty spurge, *Euphorbia peplus*, are the commonest species.

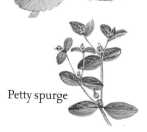

Sun spurge

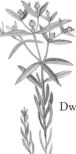

Dwarf spurge

Petty spurge

Wood-sorrel

Oxalis acetosella

Widespread and common throughout the British Isles in woods and other shady places. A low, creeping plant, 5–15 cm (2–6 inches) high. Leaves shamrock-shaped, and lime green when young. Flowers April to May, five white petals on a delicate stem.

Wood-sorrel is a plant principally of ancient deciduous woods, but it can tolerate the shade and acid soils of evergreen plantations better than many species, and often survives coniferisation. On the otherwise dark and barren floors the leaves of the wood-sorrel can appear an almost luminous viridian. They lie in scattered clusters amongst the needles, like fretwork. Gerard Manley Hopkins described the new leaves as having the sharp appearance of green lettering. They are folded to begin with, in the shape of an episcopal hat, then open flat, three hearts with their points joined at the stem.

The leaves of wood-sorrel have an agreeably sharp, fruity taste, a little like the skins of young grapes, and they were in use as a salad vegetable certainly as early as the fourteenth century. By the fifteenth century wood-sorrel was under cultivation, and in the seventeenth John Evelyn recommended it in a list of plants suitable for the kitchen garden.

Its use then was as an ingredient for salads, or pulped with sugar as a sauce for meat and fish. It can be used the same way today, but sparingly, since it contains certain oxalates which are not too good for the body in large quantities. It is these salts which are responsible for the plant's pleasantly sharp taste.

In the United States, other members of the Oxalis family (such as the yellow-flowered Oxalis stricta) are widely used, especially as flavourings for cakes.

· ·

Jewel-weed, Orange Balsam

Impatiens capensis

The jewel-weed or orange balsam is an increasingly frequent plant along the banks of rivers and canals in the south of England. It can often form magnificent bushes, up to 120 cm (4 ft) high and festooned with mottled orange nasturtium-like bells.

Jewel-weed is an introduction from North America and was not found in the wild in this country until 1822. In its native land the young leaves and stems were used as a vegetable. The green seed-pods and seeds of another immigrant balsam, the Himalayan balsam (*Impatiens glandulifera*) are also eaten in their native Asian habitats. They make a refreshingly nutty snack.

. . . .

Sea-holly
Eryngium maritimum

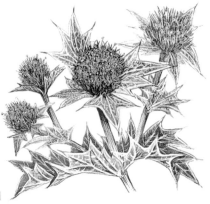

Locally common on sandy and shingle beaches. A thistle-like perennial, 20–60 cm (8–24 inches) high, with spiny, ice-blue leaves covered with bloom and ribbed and edged with a fine white tracery of veins. Flowers blue, in rounded heads with spiny bracts, June to August.

A beautiful plant of the seashore which has suffered much for the sake of holidaymakers' vases. Sea-holly likes the rough ground of sandy and shingle beaches, and its roots have consequently been confused more than once with those of the vitriolic horned-poppy.

Sea-holly roots, known as eryngo roots, were once extensively used for making candied sweetmeats. The roots – which could be up to 2 m (6 ft) long – were dug up in the spring or autumn, partly boiled until they could be peeled and then cut into thin slices. These were cooked with an equal weight of sugar until the latter became syrup, when the roots were removed and allowed to cool. Candied eryngo roots were a vital ingredient of that redoubtable Elizabethan dish, marrow-bone pie. They were also roasted, when they acquired something of the flavour of chestnuts.

Note that under the Wildlife and Countryside Act it is now illegal to dig up wild plants by the root, except on your own land, or with the permission of the landowner.

. . . .

Cow Parsley

Anthriscus sylvestris

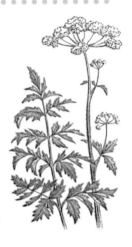

Widespread and abundant on footpaths, roadsides, banks etc. An erect, leafy, branched perennial, usually about 1 m (3 ft) high, with hollow, green, furrowed stems, hairy near the bottom of the plant but smooth above. The leaves are grass-green, slightly downy, and much divided, resembling wedge-shaped ferns. Umbels of tiny white flowers, April to June.

No plant shapes our roadside landscape more than cow parsley. In May its lacy white flowers teem along every path and hedgebank. It grows prolifically; road verges can be blanketed with it for miles on end, and can be broadened several feet by its overhanging foliage.

Yet it has been almost totally overlooked as a herb, even though one of its less common names is wild chervil. It is in fact the closest wild relative of cultivated chervil (*Anthriscus cerefolium*) a little coarser than that garden variety, maybe, but sharing the same fresh, spicy flavour.

Cow parsley is the first common umbellifer to come into flower in the spring, and this is often enough to identify it positively. But since there are a number of related species which resemble it, and which can cause serious poisoning, I have included below some notes on the characteristics which unequivocally identify cow parsley. The most dangerous sources of confusion are fool's parsley (see p. 139) and hemlock (p. 141).

Cow parsley grows up to 1.2 m (4 ft) tall, and never as high as hemlock, which can reach 2.1 m (7 ft) or more. Fool's parsley is an altogether more flimsy shrub, rarely exceeding 30 cm (1 ft). Cow parsley's stem is stout, furrowed and slightly hairy, as against hemlock's purple-spotted stems and the thin, hairless, stems of fool's parsley. In addition, hemlock has an offensive, mousy smell when any part of it is bruised, and fool's parsley has unmistakable drooping green bracts beneath the flower-heads, giving them a rather bearded appearance. Note, however, that these few pointers are in no way a substitute for a well-illustrated field guide; they are merely intended to bring out the most prominent and useful differentiating characteristics.

You should pick cow parsley as soon as the stems are sufficiently developed for you to identify it. Later in the year it becomes rather bitter. It dries well, so pick enough to last you through the off-season as well as for your immediate needs. But do not gather the plant from the sides of major roads, where it will have been contaminated by car exhausts.

Chervil is a very versatile herb, and small quantities make a lively addition to most sorts of salads, particularly cold potato, tomato and cucumber. It also makes a good flavouring for hot haricot beans, and, with chopped chives, tarragon and parsley, the famous *omelette aux fines herbes*.

A second crop of non-flowering leaves often appears in the autumn and remains green throughout the winter, and those experienced enough to tell the plant from its leaves alone could do worse than pick some fresh for winter soups and casseroles. It goes well with hot baked potatoes, and as an addition to the French country dish cassoulet.

Species	Size	Stem
Cow parsley	up to 1.2 m (4 ft)	Stout, pale green, furrowed, slightly hairy
Fool's parsley	up to 0.5 m (1 ½ ft)	Thin, hairless, ribbed
Hemlock	up to 2.1 m (7 ft)	Stout, smooth, purple-spotted

Sweet Cicely

Myrrhis odorata

Quite common on waysides and stream banks in the north of England and Scotland. An aromatic, hairy, branched perennial which grows to 1–1.5 m (4–5 ft). Leaves elegant, feathery, aniseed-scented when crushed. Large umbels of white flowers, May to July.

Cicely is one of the few plants where the connotation 'sweet' refers as much to taste as to scent. The feathery leaves have distinctly sugary overtones to their mild aniseed flavour, and are ideal for flavouring stewed fruits such as gooseberries and plums.

The species was probably introduced to Britain by the Romans, and in some places it is still known as the 'Roman plant'. It is now widely naturalised in northern Britain, and makes a handsome show on roadsides against a backdrop of drystone walls. The sixteenth-century herbalist Gerard was a great fan, and recommended both the roots (boiled) and the leaves (in salads). But he regarded the seeds as the plant's choicest part: 'Eaten as a sallad whilest they are yet greene, with oyle, vinegar and pepper, they exceed all other sallads by many degrees, both in pleasantness of taste, sweetnesse of smell, and wholesomeness for the cold and feeble stomack.'

The long green seeds can be eaten straight from the plant in June. They are up to 2.5 cm (1 inch) long and resemble miniature gherkins. Their crisp texture and sweet-and-sour aniseed taste make them an excellent wayside nibble, or an excellent foil to bread and cheese on a picnic.

In France, the young leaf-sprays are dipped in batter and fried as an hors d'oeuvre. Sweet cicely is also one of the herbs used in the making of Chartreuse, and in Cumbria the leaves were once used to polish oak doors.

Coriander
Coriandrum sativum

Short, hairless annual, up to 50 cm (20 inches) tall, bearing white flowers which appear in June to August. Fruit red-brown, ridged, aromatic when crushed.

When you come across a green coriander plant, it is difficult to believe that it will eventually produce those warmly aromatic seeds that are used so extensively in curries. The flavour of the green leaves is strong, slightly soapy and reminiscent of rue. But the smell and taste can grow on you, and the leaves are popular additions to Mediterranean salads and stews.

Coriander was probably brought to the British Isles from its native Mediterranean habitat by the Romans, and it is naturalised here in a few scattered places on waste ground. The dried seeds are mentioned in Exodus and are one of the oldest-known spices. Ground up, they are an essential ingredient of most curries, and will add a subtle flavour to soups, and, above all, to pork dishes. Len Deighton's recommendation: 'Hurl crushed coriander seeds into any open pot you see.'

* *

Alexanders

Smyrnium olustratum

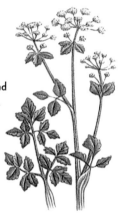

Widespread and locally abundant in hedgebanks and waste places, especially near the sea. A bushy, solid-stemmed hairless plant growing up to 120 cm (4 ft) high. Leaves glossy, toothed, in groups of three at the end of the leaf stalk, the other end being joined to the main stem by a substantial sheath. Umbels of yellow-green flowers, April to June.

The Romans brought alexanders to this country from the Mediterranean, as a pot-herb – the 'parsley of Alexandria'. It thrived, became naturalised, and was still being planted in kitchen gardens in the early eighteenth century.

Today it is widely naturalised in hedgebanks near the coast. It sprouts early and rapidly in the spring, and its bright, glossy leaves can sometimes be seen pushing through January snows.

The young leaves make a spicy addition to salads, and the flower-buds can be pickled, but the most succulent part of the plant is the stem. You should cut those leaf stems which grow near the base of the plant, where they are thick and have been partially blanched by the surrounding grass or the plant's own foliage. You should be able to cut about 15 cm (6 inches) of pinkish stalk from each stem (discarding the greener bits). Don't be put off by the plant's rather cloying angelica smell; this disappears almost completely with cooking.

Cooked alexanders

Cook the stems in boiling water for not more than 10 minutes. Then eat them like asparagus, with molten butter. They have a delicate texture, and a pleasantly aromatic taste.

Pignut
Conopodium majus

Occurs on well-drained soils in grassland and woodland. A slender, single-stemmed perennial, 20–80 cm (8–32 inches) high. Leaves feathery with narrow lobes. Flowers white, in dense, flat heads, May to July.

This slender, feathery umbellifer is still common in June and July in woods, meadows and sandy heaths, but of course it is now illegal to dig it up except on your own land. Once, pignuts (or earth nuts) were one of the most popular of children's wayside nibbles, even though extracting them from the ground was as delicate a business as an egg and spoon race. They cannot be pulled out, for the thin leaf stalk breaks off very quickly. The fine white roots must be unearthed with a knife, and carefully traced down to the tuber, which lies about 10–20 cm (4–8 inches) below the surface.

The roundish 'nuts', dark brown and the size of walnuts, can be eaten raw, once they have been scraped or washed, and taste somewhere between hazelnuts and celery. One early botanist recommended them peeled and boiled in broth with pepper. They were also added to stews, when the taste reputedly becomes more like parsnip. Pignuts are worth trying if you have legal access to the roots.

. . . .

Ground-elder, Goutweed

Aegopodium podagraria

Widespread and common in shady places on waste ground, under hedges, in gardens, throughout Europe. A perennial forming large patches 30–100 cm (1–3 ft) high. Leaves finely toothed, in groups of three at the end of the leaf stems. Flowers June to August, white umbels on a hairless stem.

Though no relation of the elder, goutweed's leaves do bear a superficial resemblance to those of the common and similarly prolific tree. It can often be found in quite large patches by roadsides and under garden hedges, its pale green leaves making a bright carpet in the shady places. Its continued presence in both habitats is a telling example of the persistence of some weeds in places where they were once cultivated and valued.

Ground elder was probably introduced to Britain by the Romans. In the Middle Ages it was grown in gardens as a vegetable, and at roadside inns and monasteries as a supposed quick palliative for travellers' gout. Advances in medical understanding put paid to the second of these functions, and the growing preference for milder-tasting, fuller-leaved vegetables to the first. Any popularity ground elder still retained was finally undermined by the imperialistic tendencies of its rootstock, which would quickly take over its host's garden. Even in the sixteenth century, when the plant was still being used as a pot-herb, John Gerard wrote complainingly of it that 'once taken roote, it will hardly be gotten out again, spoiling and getting every yeere more ground, to the annoying of better herbes' – a sentiment which many modern gardeners will echo. In fact, one way of getting back at the invader is to eat it. Cooked like a spinach, for about five minutes, it makes an unusual vegetable. Its tangy, aromatic flavour, though, is not to everyone's taste, so it is as well to try it in small quantities first.

Rock Samphire
Crithmum maritimum

Frequent on rocky coasts in the south and west. A squat, bushy plant growing up to 30 cm (1 ft) high. Stems hairless and solid, leaves fleshy, grey-green and cut into narrow untoothed leaflets. Flowers are yellow umbels, July to October.

A plant of rocky coasts, occasionally on shingle, and you might catch the warm but slightly sulphurous smell of rock samphire before you see it. Both stems and leaves can be used, but before cooking remove any leaves that have begun to turn slimy, and any hard parts of the stalk. Then boil in water for about ten minutes, and serve with melted butter. To eat, suck the fleshy parts away from the stringy veins.

Rock samphire pickle

Soak the samphire in water for 2–3 hours, drain and then cook briefly in wine vinegar, water and salt. Cool and store in jars with fresh vinegar, water and salt so it remains green.

Rock samphire hash

This curious recipe dates from the mid seventeenth century. This sauce was used as a garnish for meat, and the whole dish dressed with fresh samphire leaves and bright red barberries.

100 g (4 oz) samphire, chopped
1 handful diced pickled cucumber and capers
500 ml (1 pint) stock
2 tablespoons wine vinegar
1 lemon
Slivers of butter
1 egg yolk
Pepper and nutmeg to taste

1 Mix the chopped samphire with the pickled cucumbers and capers.
2 Mix the stock with the wine vinegar, the juice and grated peel of the lemon, and pepper and nutmeg. Bring to the boil and then add the samphire. Simmer for half an hour.
3 Take off the boil and gradually add slivers of butter and the egg yolk, stirring constantly until the mixture thickens.

The Water-dropworts

Oenanthe species

☠️ **POISONOUS**

Responsible for the majority of fatalities from wild plant poisoning in this country – often from European visitors mistaking the roots for parsnips, etc. All species – including tubular water-dropwort (O. fistulosa) fine-leaved water-dropwort (O. aquatica) and parsley water-dropwort (O. lachenalii) – are deadly poisonous, often rapidly and suddenly.

The commonest and most widespread species is hemlock water-dropwort (*Oenanthe crocata*). It is widespread and locally common in or by fresh water. A stout, hairless plant, up to 120 cm (4 ft) high, often forming clumps. The stem is usually hollow, and the foliage glossy, divided and smelling pleasantly of parsley. Flowers June to August, large white umbels.

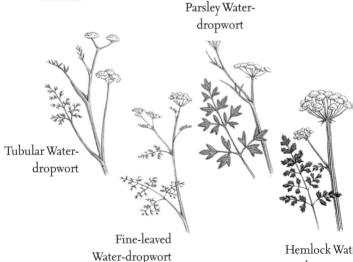

Parsley Water-dropwort

Tubular Water-dropwort

Fine-leaved Water-dropwort

Hemlock Water-dropwort

Fool's Parsley

Aethusa cynapium

☠ **POISONOUS**

A low, weak, hairless annual, often growing
as a weed in gardens and other cultivated
ground. Parsley-like foliage, and flowers in
white umbels, over a distinctive ring of bracts which
makes them look bearded. The plant has a distasteful smell which
puts off most pickers, but poisoning has occasionally occurred. It is
rarely fatal in healthy subjects.

Fennel

Foeniculum vulgare

Locally distributed throughout the
south of England, Midlands, East
Anglia and Wales. Less common in
the north and Scotland. Occurs on
cliffs, waste ground and damp places,
especially near the sea. Tall, greyish
perennial to 2 m (6 ft). Leaves threadlike and
aromatic. Flowers early June to October; clusters
of mustard-yellow blossoms.

See fennel's feathery sprays along damp coastal roadsides in
early July, and you will understand the attraction it held for
the early herbalists. Its umbels of yellow flowers and
smooth, threadlike leaves are elegantly soft, giving the plant
a curiously foppish air beside the hairy yokels it shares its
living space with. Crush the leaves in your hand and they

give off a powerful aromatic odour, reminiscent of aniseed. On a hot summer's day this is enough to betray the plant's presence, for the cool tang stands out from the heavy, sweet musk of hogweed and elder like a throwback to a sharp April morning.

Fennel was probably introduced to Britain by the Romans, and it now occurs throughout the southern half of the country, on cliffs as much as on roadsides, but it tends to grow in rather localised patches. All parts of the plant are edible, from the stalks – if your teeth are strong enough – to the rather sparse bulb. (The larger fennel bulbs available in the shops belong to cultivated Florence fennel, *Foeniculum vulgare* var. *dulce*.) They all have a fresh, nutty flavour. But it is the thinner stalks, leaf-sprays and seeds that are the most useful.

The green parts of the plant should be cut with a sharp knife early in the summer, and some (stalks included) hung up to dry for the winter. Fennel smells stronger as it dries, and after a few weeks a good-sized bunch will be powerful enough to scent a whole room. The seeds should be gathered late in October, just before they are fully dry.

Fennel leaves are popular in cooking, particularly in fish dishes, though the tradition of using it in this way probably derives from nothing more than the plant's preference for coastal areas. Gooseberry and fennel sauce is a classic accompaniment for mackerel (see p. 107). The dried stalks form the basis of the famous Provençal red mullet dish, *rouget flambé au fenouil*. The finely chopped green leaves are also good to add to liver, potato salad, parsnips, and even, Len Deighton recommends, apple pie.

Fennel was one of the Anglo-Saxon herbalists' nine sacred herbs, and the seeds were valued as – among other things – a remedy for wind. The digestive properties of the seeds are still recognised, and they are sometimes served at the end of Indian meals.

Okrochka

This exotic cold soup from the near East makes use of the cool fragrance of fennel. It is a perfect dish on a warm summer evening, and utilises some other wild summer herbs you may gather.

250 ml (10 fl oz) yoghurt (natural or apple)
250 ml (10 fl oz) milk
1 cup diced fresh cucumber
1/2 cup chopped pickled cucumber or gherkin
1/2 cup diced cooked chicken
1 handful finely chopped fennel leaves
Fresh summer herbs (e.g. mint, parsley, chives)
2 hard-boiled eggs, chopped
Salt and pepper to taste

1 Mix the yoghurt and milk in a good-sized bowl.
2 Add the fresh cucumber, pickled cucumber or gherkin, chicken and fennel together with a little of the other summer herbs.
3 Season with salt and pepper and put in the fridge for at least two hours.
4 Before serving, add the roughly chopped hard-boiled eggs, and sprinkle the surface with a little more black pepper and fresh herbs.

• •

Hemlock

Conium maculataum

☠ POISONOUS

Common on waste ground and by streams. Flowers June, July, in white umbels. A tall plant, up to 2.1 m (7 ft) high, with feathery foliage

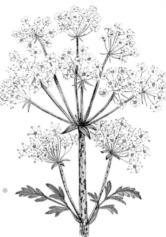

and hollow, purple-spotted stems. The whole plant emits an unpleasant mousy odour when bruised. Most toxic when young and green, and the poisonous alkaloids are destroyed by drying and heat.

· ·

Wild Celery

Apium graveolens

Widespread but local in damp places near the sea, and mainly in the south and east of England. Flowers June to September. A strongly smelling plant, growing about 30–60 cm (1–2 ft) high, with shiny, yellow-green leaves, shaped much like those of garden celery, and rather sparse white umbels of flowers.

The powerful aroma of wild celery, or smallage, largely disappears on drying, leaving a herb which is exactly like strong celery in flavour, and ideal for soups. To make a straight cream of wild celery – much richer and tangier than garden celery soup – pick a small bunch of the leaves, dry for about three weeks (in a little-used room), then simmer for about half an hour in some chicken stock. Strain, stir in a cupful of hot milk and serve immediately.

But even in the fresh, undried state, the taste is nothing like as powerful as might be expected. The stems are not of course as bity as those of the garden variety, but I have found that a few of them, chopped, make a brisk ingredient for salads.

Parsley

Petroselinum crispum

**A sturdy plant of sandy and rocky banks,
similar to the familiar garden herb, but
lacking its thick, feathery leaf clusters.**

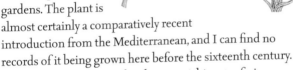

It is doubtful whether any of the
parsley plants which
can occasionally be
found growing wild
on rocky places near
the sea are any more
than escapees from
gardens. The plant is
almost certainly a comparatively recent
introduction from the Mediterranean, and I can find no
records of it being grown here before the sixteenth century.

As a change from a redundant garnishing, try frying
parsley for half a minute in hot butter and serving it as a
vegetable with fish. It is extremely rich in vitamin C.

Scots Lovage

Ligusticum scoticum

**A stocky umbellifer, 60–90 cm (2–3 ft), with bright green, leathery
leaves, which grows locally on rocky sea cliffs in Scotland. It was
occasionally eaten against scurvy.**

Its cultivated cousin, *Levisticum officinale*, is naturalised from
herb gardens in a few places. This domesticated lovage is a

much more distinctive plant, growing over 3.5 m (11–12 ft) tall, and its uses are correspondingly wider. The hollow stems have been candied like angelica, and blanched like celery for use as a salad vegetable.

The flavour of both varieties is curious, basically resembling celery, but having quite strong yeasty overtones. Because of this lovage has been used to add body to the flavour of soups and casseroles when meat is short.

Lovage is scarce in the wild, and the best way of experiencing its flavour may be to grow *Levisticum officinale* in the herb garden – though it is a very large perennial.

Wild Parsnip

Pastinaca sativa

A native umbellifer of chalk and limestone in the southeast of England. In the poor soils of road verges and waste ground it often grows to no more than 45 cm (18 inches) in height.

The wild parsnip is a stocky, economical plant, with none of the excess and luxuriance of some of our Umbelliferae. Its chrome-yellow umbels could only really be confused with those of fennel, but it lacks the feathery leaves and aniseed smell. *Pastinaca sativa* is almost certainly an ancestor of our cultivated parsnips. An experiment in Cirencester in the mid nineteenth century produced large, fleshy roots from the wild stock in ten years. No more was done than to transplant the wild parsnips into rich garden soil, and resow each season with the seeds of those specimens with the largest roots.

Cultivation of this kind was almost certainly under way in the Middle Ages, as the parsnip was valued as a sweetening ingredient for sauces, cakes and puddings. The wild roots are just about edible after the first frosts but they are thin and wiry and of more historical than culinary interest.

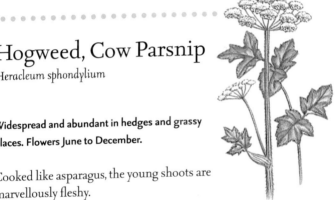

Hogweed, Cow Parsnip
Heracleum sphondylium

Widespread and abundant in hedges and grassy places. Flowers June to December.

Cooked like asparagus, the young shoots are marvellously fleshy.

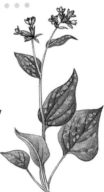

Lungwort
Pulmonaria officinalis

An intriguing flower, somewhat similar to the closely related comfrey, except that its leaves are covered with a rash of white spots.

Lungwort is a frequent escape from gardens,

where it used to be grown as a medicine 'gainst the infirmities and ulcers of the lungs'. Gerard also recommends it as a boiled vegetable.

. . . .

Common Comfrey

Symphytum officinale

Widespread and common in ditches and by riverbanks throughout the British Isles. A bushy, hairy perennial, growing up to 120 cm (4 ft) high, with dark green spear-shaped leaves. Flowers June to October, white, cream, mauve or pink bells in clusters.

Comfrey is an increasingly common plant of damp places, especially by running water. In this sort of habitat its broad, spear-shaped leaves are unmistakable, even when the plant is not in bloom. They are dull and hairy underneath, a fine, dark, almost glossy green above, and with slightly indented reticulations, as if the leaves had been pressed against a mould.

It is the leaves which are now used in cookery. Don't worry about their furry texture; this disappears completely during cooking. Nor is there much need to be particular about the age of the leaves you use, for in my experience the older ones (provided of course they have not started to wither) have more flavour than the younger. One way of using them is to boil them like spinach, with plenty of seasoning. There is no need to add butter, as the leaves themselves are fairly glutinous. The young leaf spears, picked in March when they are no more than a couple of centimetres tall, make excellent salads, not unlike sliced cucumber.

Comfrey (from the Latin *confervere*, to grow together) was the medieval herbalists' favourite bone-setter. The root was lifted in the spring, grated up and used as plaster is today. In a short while the mash would set as solid as a hard wood. In fact the whole plant was one of those 'wonder herbs' that was used for every sort of knitting operation from drawing splinters to healing ruptures. Gerard's recommendation was even more eclectic:

'The slimie substance of the roote made in a posset of ale, and given to drinke against the paine in the backe, gotten by any violent motion, as wrestling, or over much use of women, doth in fower or five daies perfectly cure the same.'

Schwarzwurz

The best recipe for comfrey leaves is this Teutonic fritter. They make an excellent companion to fried fish, which echo the shape of the leaves.

Comfrey leaves, as many as required
1 egg
50 g (2 oz) plain flour
250 ml (½ pint) milk or water
½ teaspoon sea salt. Butter or oil for frying

1 Leave the stalks on the comfrey leaves, wash well, and dip into a thin batter made from the egg, flour, milk or water and salt.
2 Fry the battered leaf in oil for no more than two minutes.
3 For a more succulent result stick two or three similarly-sized leaves together before battering.
The crisp golden batter contrasts delightfully with the mild, glutinous leaves.

Borage
Borago officinalis

Quite common as an escape on waysides and waste places. A loosely bushy annual, 30–60 cm (1–2 ft) with conspicuously hairy stems, leaves and sepals. Flowers bright blue, with reflexed petals and prominent purple stamens, May to September.

Borage once had a great reputation as a sort of herbal pep-pill. It was renowned as an aphrodisiac and as a general dispeller of melancholy and depression. John Evelyn clearly understood the type of person who would perennially be in need of such aids when he wrote that 'the sprigs ... are of known virtue to revive the hypochondriac and cheer the hard student'.

Whatever its medicinal qualities, the young leaves and bright blue, star-like flowers make a refreshing and fragrant addition to claret cups and other summer drinks, particularly in combination with woodruff. The star-shaped petals look appealing floated out on top of the drink – or frozen inside ice cubes. In more leisurely days, Richard Jeffries noted in *Nature Near London* (1883), borage leaves used 'to float in the claret cup ladled out to thirsty travellers at the London railway stations'.

Oysterplant
Mertensia maritima

A hairless perennial of shingle beaches, with reddish trailing stems and fleshy, blue-green leaves. Flowers in clusters, pink turning blue, June to August.

This is a rare plant that grows on a few stretches of coastal shingle in Scotland, in prostrate mats. The fleshy leaves have been eaten both raw and cooked, and taste like oysters.

. . . .

Dead-nettles

The young shoots and leaves of these common and familiar weeds can be added to salads, stir-fried as a green vegetable (either by themselves or in company with other spring greens), or washed and cooked with no additional water but with a knob of butter, salt and pepper and some chopped spring onions, for about ten minutes. Finish with a dash of lemon juice or a sprinkling of nutmeg.

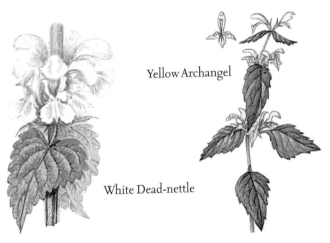

Yellow Archangel

White Dead-nettle

Yellow Archangel
Lamiastrum galeobdolon

Widespread and locally common in old woodland and shady hedgerows in England and Wales. Flowers May to June.

White Dead-nettle

Lamium album

Widespread and common in hedgebanks, waste places and gardens. Rare and local in the north and west of Scotland, and in the west of Ireland. Flowers March to November.

Red Dead-nettle

Lamium purpureum

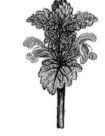

Widespread and abundant in cultivated ground throughout the British Isles. Flowers throughout the year in mild conditions.

Henbit Dead-nettle

Lamium amplexicaule

Locally common in cultivated ground, commonest in the east of Britain. Flowers March to October.

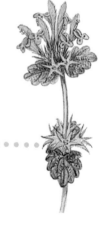

. . . .

Ground-ivy
Glechoma hederacea

Common in woods, hedges, cultivated ground. A low, creeping perennial, often carpeting the ground. Leaves kidney-shaped, long-stalked, softly hairy. Flowers blue, in whorls at the base of the leaves, March to June.

The dried leaves of ground-ivy make one of the more

agreeable herbal teas, cooling and with a sharp, slight fragrance. Before hops became widely accepted in the seventeenth century, ground-ivy – known then as alehoof – was one of the chief agents for flavouring and clarifying ale. In the seventeenth century, Nicholas Culpeper wrote of it:

'It is good to tun up with new drink, for it will clarify it in a night, that it will be fitter to be dranke the next morning; or if any drinke be thick with removing or any other accident, it will do the like in a few hours.'

Balm
Melissa officinalis

Naturalised in hedgebanks and shady places in southern England. A medium hairy perennial with yellow-green pointed leaves. Flowers white or pale yellow in leafy whorls, July to September.

A Mediterranean herb, introduced and widely naturalised in waste places and near gardens in the south of England. Balm is an undistinguished-looking plant like a bushy mint, yet it has always been popular in herb gardens. Bees adore the flowers, and it was reputed that they would never leave a garden that had a clump of balm growing. While a beehive was still a standard fixture in gardens, so was a 'bee-balm'.

Balm is still grown for its strongly lemon-scented leaves, which make a refreshing tea. The leaves can also be added to wine-cups, or they can act as a substitute for lemons in stuffings and salads, and can be used to give a tang to apple jelly.

Lemon-balm tea

Make an infusion of fresh leaves and stalks, strain and drink as it is. Or add ice to make a cooler for hot days. Fresh or dried leaves can also be added to light Indian or China teas for extra flavour and for their medicinal effects. It has a gentle calming action that can relieve tension.

Wild Marjoram, Oregano
Origanum vulgare

Widespread and locally common in grassy places on chalk and limestone. Rare in Scotland. A slender herb, growing up to 1 m (3 ft) high, with downy stems extensively branched near the top of the plant. The leaves are oval and usually untoothed, and the flowers a pale, pinkish purple, in bunches at the head of the plant. Flowers July to October.

The marjoram growing wild in Britain is also known as the herb oregano. It is spicier than sweet marjoram, Origanum majorana (the herb marjoram, a more southern species). Oregano is one of the elemental flavours of Mediterranean cooking. It belongs with the pervasive mixture of tomato and garlic and olive oil and adds a warm, earthy fragrance that seems to capture the essence of the hot south. In Britain, marjoram never achieves quite the rough fragrance it does in sunnier parts. However, gathered in summer it is perfect for drying, and used in winter it recalls something of the spirit of warmer months.

When you find marjoram growing wild on a dry heath or chalky roadside bank, its flimsy, slightly grey-tinted leaves look very appetising, and used raw they do indeed make a pleasantly pungent addition to salads. For use as a herb, pick some sprigs of the plant, flowers and all, whilst it is in full bloom, and later strip off the leaves and blossoms from the rather wiry stalk. But be on the watch for discoloured or 'burnt' leaves. The plant is prone to moulds and rusts, and infected leaves, though harmless, are usually musty to taste.

Oregano is above all a meat herb. It gives a fine savour to stews and casseroles, to spaghetti sauces and shepherd's pie, even to grilled steaks, if they are first rubbed with the herb. But wild marjoram becomes sweeter as it dries, and can then be used in a wider range of dishes. In the south of England tea made from marjoram leaves used to be popular, and large quantities were gathered and hung up to dry. Marjoram has also been used for medicinal purposes since ancient times, either as an infusion or in oil.

Olives oregano

When olives are steeped in a marinade of oil flavoured with the freshly picked plant, they acquire something of the aroma of the herb. To 500 g (1 lb) of pricked olives in a jar, add one cup of olive oil, one teaspoon of thyme, one teaspoon of crushed peppercorns and three teaspoons of chopped wild marjoram. Close the jar, shake well and leave in a refrigerator for at least two days. Olives treated like this make a perfect centrepiece for a lunch for the season when marjoram is in flower. Serve them with a light red wine and cheese.

Marjoram sugar

Add chopped flowers, buds and a few young leaves to a jar of caster sugar, and stand in the sun for a day. The scent will subtly transfer to the sugar, which can then used for sprinkling on cake, fruit and desserts.

Herb scones

These unusual scones should be served with roast meat or vegetables.

50 g (2 oz) butter
100 g (4 oz) salted flour
1 heaped teaspoon chopped marjoram

1 Rub the butter into the flour until it resembles breadcrumbs.
2 Add the marjoram, and enough cold water to make a stiff dough. Mix well but lightly with a knife, and then shape into thin cakes with your hands.
3 Put them on a greased tray in the oven for 12–15 minutes (longer if you are cooking the meat slowly).

Wild Thyme
Thymus polytrichus

Widespread and often abundant in grassy places, especially on chalk and limestone, and on sandy heaths. A prostrate,

creeping plant, with rather woody stems and runners, 5–10 cm (2–4 inches). Leaves very small, oval, and ranged in many opposing pairs along the stalks. The flowers are reddish purple in roundish bunches at the ends of the stalks, June to August.

Wild thyme is one of the most pleasantly scented of herbs. But be under no illusion: your nostrils are not going to be filled with that heady aroma as you stride over the springy turf with your basket. Wild thyme has neither the bushy forthrightness nor the pungency of cultivated thyme (Thymus vulgaris) or of the species that grow so conspicuously in the Mediterranean. It is a subtle, skulking plant, often growing entirely below grass level. Finding it is a hands-and-knees job, a rummage through the miniature downland flora, the milkworts and violets, for a sprig of toy, oval leaves that yield that clovy smell between the fingers. Then, tracing the runners back, following their meanderings through the dry lower stems of the grasses back to the woody root.

For a short while, when each plant is in flower, picking is a simpler exercise – though less rewarding I think than the fingertip ferreting for the spring and autumn shoots. The flower-heads are large compared to the size of the plant and, like marjoram, conspicuous for their attendant insects. Wild thyme is best picked when in full bloom, so that the honey-scented flowers can be used as well as the leaves.

If you like you can strip the leaves and flowers off the stalk before using. But as wild thyme is considerably milder than the garden variety you can afford to use large sprigs of it liberally – and indeed to try it out in unconventional combinations. The great virtue of wild thyme is precisely its versatility.

Try it as a tea, or chopped finely and beaten into butter. Add it to omelettes and to stuffings for roast chicken. But think of it, too, as a convenient way of perking up picnic or outdoor food. A few sprigs can be added to pots of cottage cheese, tucked inside sandwiches, thrown into almost any casserole and wrapped up with roast joints in foil. In Scandinavia, steeped in aquavit, it makes one of the favourite varieties of schnapps.

Thyme soup

Patience Gray has a simple but comforting Catalan shepherd's recipe in her classic book Honey From a Weed. Soak several slices of dry white bread in olive oil. Infuse a bunch of dried wild thyme in boiling water for five minutes, then pour this over the oily bread and serve.

- -

Water Mint

Mentha aquatica

Widespread and common by the edges of streams, in damp meadows and woods, throughout the British Isles. A rough, hairy mint, often growing in quite sizeable clumps up to 60 cm (2 ft) high. The leaves are frequently tinged with purple, and grow in opposed pairs. Bluish-lilac flowers chiefly in a round bushy head at the top of the plant, July to September.

Water mint can be used exactly as if it were a garden mint. Try adding mint to your cooked egg and cheese dishes, as well as to peas and potatoes. But if you should find the taste of water mint a little too bitter, even in a well-sugared mint sauce, try the recipe for Indian mint chutney, in which the wild mint's sharper qualities can be a positive virtue. Alternatively, add a few sprigs to a pot of China tea, or make a simple mint tea by steeping the leaves in hot (not boiling) water for about five minutes.

Mint chutney

50 g (2 oz) mint leaves, 2 tablespoons vinegar
100 g (4 oz) tamarind, chopped
50 g (2 oz) green chillies
1 onion, 1 clove of garlic
1 dessertspoon salt

1 Wash and dry the mint, and grind (or liquidise) to a thick paste with the vinegar.
2 Add the tamarind, chillies, onion, garlic and salt to the mint paste and mix thoroughly.
3 Bottle and store for a few days before using.

There are over a dozen varieties of mint growing either wild or naturalised in Britain. All can be used more or less like water mint, though the quality of their flavours varies. The following are the most frequently found.

Corn Mint

Mentha arvensis

Widespread and frequent in arable land, heaths, damp woodland rides. A much-maligned plant whose fragrance has been described as 'acrid' by one writer, like 'wet mouldy gorgonzola' by Geoffrey Grigson, but as 'a strong fulsome mixed smell of mellow apples and gingerbread' by the eighteenth-century mint expert William Sole. You must judge for yourself.

Spear Mint

Mentha spicata

The mint usually grown in gardens, and frequently found naturalised near houses.

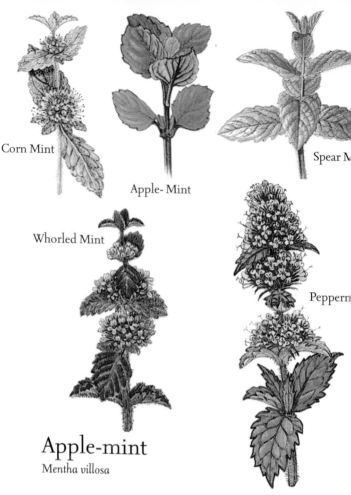

Corn Mint

Apple- Mint

Spear M

Whorled Mint

Peppern

Apple-mint
Mentha villosa

Another garden escape. Apple-scented, and good in summer drinks.

Whorled Mint
Mentha verticillata

Widespread and not uncommon in damp places. Many members of the mint family hybridise readily with each other, and this species is a cross between our two commonest mints, water mint and corn mint.

Peppermint
Mentha piperita

This mint occurs only rarely in the wild, yet it is a natural hybrid between spear mint and water mint. It was not discovered in this country until the late seventeenth century. But why peppermint? It has a sharp taste, certainly, but nothing like the fieriness of pepper. The herb is now extensively cultivated for its aromatic oil, which is used in toothpastes, sweets and indigestion remedies.

. . . .

Greater Plantain
Plantago major

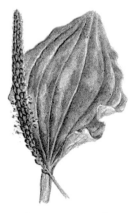

More like a grass than a flower, the greater plantain has long, pale green flower-heads, 15–45 cm (6–18 inches) high, perfectly described by their alternative name of 'rat's-tails'.

Plantain is one of those plants that positively thrive on rough treatment. The more you walk on it or mow it the better it does. The North American Indians went as far as to call it 'Englishman's foot', for wherever the white man walked and worked, plantain followed. Its rosettes of ribbed oval leaves are abundant on lawns and footpaths.

The young leaves have been used as a salad herb, but I find them too tough and bitter when raw, and would advise them to be well cooked as a spinach.

Brooklime

Veronica beccabunga

**Widespread and common by the edges of streams and
in wet places. Flowers May to September.**

A quite widely used salad plant in northern Europe,
rather bitter. The American species was once praised
by *Scientific American* as 'a salad plant equal to the water-cress.
Delightful in flavour, healthful and anti-scorbutic.'

• •

Lady's Bedstraw

Galium verum

**Widespread on dry grassland, especially chalk and limestone
near the sea. A hairy perennial, 10–120 cm (4–48 inches) high,
with narrow pointed leaves and dense clusters of yellow flowers.**

Lady's bedstraw is a feathery, insubstantial plant, whose
myriads of tiny yellow flowers smell of honey when cool
and fresh. But when the plant is dried it develops the
characteristic hay-like smell of coumarin (like woodruff,
also a member of the bedstraw family). This breaks down
to yield a powerful anticoagulant, dicoumarol, and there is
always a small quantity of this in picked specimens of the
plant. Yet lady's bedstraw also contains some chemical which
overrides this, as it is of proven value as a styptic. It was once
also used as a kind of vegetable rennet, for curdling milk
into junkets and cheese. I have never found full instructions
for this old practice, and have not yet succeeded in making
more than a thin skin of rather bitter junket with it.

Goosegrass, Cleavers

Galium aparine

Widespread and abundant in hedges, woods and cultivated ground. A straggling annual, 50–180 cm (1–6 ft), with square stems and whorls of 6–8 leaves, covered in all parts with tiny turned-down prickles. Flowers inconspicuous, white, May to June.

A great children's plant, which clings mercilessly to trousers and coats and any rough surface which brushes against it. If you look at a section of the stalk of leaf under a microscope you will see that the plant's sticking power is due to the hook-like bristles which cover every part of it. Seen like this, they look positively dangerous, and certainly not fit to eat. But look at the hooks again after the plant has been plunged into boiling water for a few seconds, and you will see that they have 'melted' and quite lost their forbidding sharpness.

Boiled as a spinach before the hard round seeds appear, goosegrass makes tolerable if stringy eating, and can, moreover, be picked through winter when few other green plants are to be found. In the seventeenth century John Evelyn recommended the young shoots in spring soups and puddings.

Few meagre weeds can have had their various parts put to so many ingenious uses. The seeds have been roasted and used as a coffee. In the green state they were used to adorn the tops of lacemakers' pins (the young seeds were pushed onto the pins to make a sort of padded head). And some books report that the prickly stems and leaves were used to strain hair out of milk.

Woodruff

Galium odoratum

Widespread and often abundant in ancient woods and hedgebanks, especially beech, and on chalk and limestone. Grows in clusters to about 30 cm (1 ft) high, with whorls of six to nine leaves at intervals up the smooth stems. Flowers small, white and four-petalled, in loose heads, April to June.

In the late spring, the edges of beech woods are often thickly carpeted with the young shoots of woodruff, immaculate in their tiny marble-white flowers and brisk green ruffs. When they are green the plants are almost odourless; but allow them to dry and they quickly develop the cool, fresh smell of new-mown hay. Indeed, the plant was once popular for scenting dried linen and laying in beds.

This smell, which you will recognise if you have dried meadowsweet or melilot, is due to a chemical called coumarin (see lady's bedstraw, p. 160). The scent readily transfers to liquids, and makes dried woodruff an ideal herb to add to summer wine cups. A bottle of pure apple juice in which a sprig has been allowed to steep for a week becomes positively ambrosial.

Maibowle

The classic woodruff recipe is for *Maibowle* or *Maiwein*, traditionally drunk in Germany on May Day. Steep a bunch of dried woodruff in a jug of Moselle wine. Add a couple of tablespoons of sugar dissolved in water. Chill, and serve with thinly sliced orange.

Common Cornsalad, Lamb's-lettuce

Valerianella locusta

Quite common in arable ground, on banks and walls. A slender annual, 5–20 cm (2–8 inches). Flowers tiny, lilac, in flat-topped clusters, April to August.

A diminutive and rather bland plant that is nevertheless a useful addition to salads, especially as it stays in leaf for most of the winter. Lamb's lettuce and its cultivated cousins are popular in France, where they are known as *mache* and *salade de prêtre*. The leaves are best served with a sharp dressing to bring out their flavour and texture.

. . . .

Red Valerian

Centranthus ruber

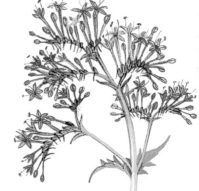

Local on walls, old buildings, wasteland and cliffs. A blue-green, hairless perennial, 30–80 cm (1–3 ft), with small red, pink or white flowers in branched clusters, May to September.

In France and Italy the very young leaves of this plant are sometimes boiled with butter as greens, or eaten raw in salads – though they are rather bitter used this way.

Red valerian was introduced to Britain from southern Europe in the sixteenth century, and was a great favourite of Gerard's, though he ascribed no practical uses to the plant. Its red flowers now adorn many stony and rocky places in the southwest.

Burdock

Arctium minus

Widespread and common throughout the British Isles, at the edges of woods, and on roadsides and waste ground. A stiff, bushy plant, up to 90 cm (3 ft) high, conspicuous early in the year for its large, floppy, heart-shaped leaves, and later for its stout branching stems. Flowers July to September. The flower-heads are egg-shaped and thistle-like, and turn at the fruiting stage into the well-known prickly burs.

Burdock is sometimes mistaken for rhubarb. Often there is nothing to be seen of the plant except its huge leaves draped over the ground. The parts to pick are the young leaf stems which begin to sprout round about May (after September they are too tough and stringy). The stems should be cut into 5 cm (2 inch) lengths and the hard outer peel stripped off. This will leave you with a moist core about the thickness of a pipe-cleaner. This can be chopped and used raw in salads, boiled and served with butter like asparagus, or added to meat soups. It has a flavour slightly reminiscent of new potatoes.

Burdock roots are used quite extensively in Japanese cooking. They are sliced thinly and braised with soy sauce, or wrapped in their own leaves and silver foil and roasted whole. If tempted to try this yourself, remember that the law requires you to obtain the landowner's permission before digging up any wild plant by the root.

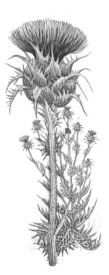

Marsh Thistle

Cirsium palustre

A tall, common thistle, up to 2 m (6 ft), found in grassy places and woods, especially on wet ground.

The young shoots have been used like burdock in some European countries. The prickles and the tough outer peel are removed, and the stalks then used in salads or boiled.

Milk Thistle

Silybum marianum

Scattered and rare in the British Isles. It is liable to spring up in any waste place, but prefers areas near the sea. A distinctive plant, growing up to 150 cm (5 ft) high. Leaves spiny, dark green, intricately veined in white. Flowers purple, June to August; flower bracts end in yellow spines.

Centuries ago this handsome thistle was introduced into western European gardens from the Mediterranean, for use as a medicinal herb. Almost all parts of the plant were eaten. The leaves were trimmed of prickles and boiled. The stems were peeled, soaked in water to remove the bitterness and then stewed like rhubarb. Even the spiny bracts that surround the broad flower-head were eaten like globe artichokes.

Hardhead, Common Knapweed
Centaurea nigra

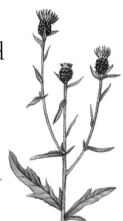

A common wayside plant, up to 1 m (3 ft), with feathery purple petals.

The petals may be used in salads, and give a splash of unusual colour if scattered over a green-leaf base.

Chicory
Cichorium intybus

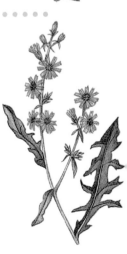

Widespread throughout England and Wales, but only locally common, usually in grassy and waste places on chalk. An untidy perennial with grooved stems, 30–120 cm (1–4 ft). Flowers pale blue, June to September.

This is the 'succory' of the old herbalists, a tall, distinguished plant with startling cornflower-blue blossoms. Chicory is probably not a native of the British Isles, but it still grows in quite a wide range of grassy habitats, especially on chalk and limestone.

The roots are boiled and eaten in the Middle East, and it is from the Arabic chicouryeh that the English name for the plant is derived. Roast and ground, the roots make an acceptable (though slightly bitter) substitute for, or addition to, coffee, and have been extensively cultivated for this purpose. Chicory was used on a wide scale during the Second World War when coffee supplies were cut off. The leaves of chicory can be used as a salad vegetable in summer, and the following five members of the daisy family can all be used similarly.

Nipplewort
Lapsana communis

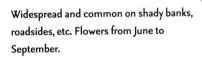

Widespread and common on shady banks, roadsides, etc. Flowers from June to September.

Cat's-ear
Hypochaeris radicata

Common in dry pastures, open woods and other grassy places. Flowers May to September, but the leaves continue to grow through much of the winter.

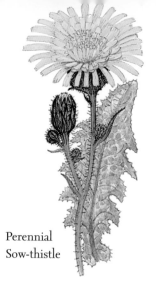

Cat's-ear

Rough Hawkbit

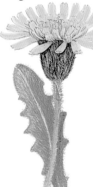

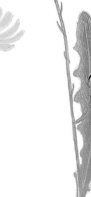

Perennial
Sow-thistle

Rough Hawkbit

Leontodon hispidus

**Common in meadows, roadside verges and dry, grassy places.
Flowers May to September.**

Perennial Sow-thistle

Sonchus arvensis

**Widespread and common throughout the British Isles, on road
verges and cultivated ground. Flowers July to October.**

Goat's-beard

Tragopogon pratensis

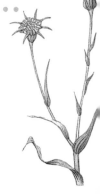

**Widespread and common in dry, grassy places.
Flowers June to September.**

Salsify

Tragopogon porrifolius

Salsify still grows wild in a few places, chiefly near estuaries in the southeast of England. It is a tall, straight plant, up to 1 m (3 ft), with purplish dandelion-like flowers.

Do not pick wild specimens whilst the plant is still so uncommon, but it ought to be purchased more often from the few shops which stock the cultivated variety. The long white roots are first carefully peeled, and then boiled or steamed with butter and lemon juice. The flavour is sufficiently individual for the roots to be served as a dish on their own.

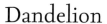

Dandelion

Taraxacum species

Widespread and abundant in open and grassy places throughout British Isles. Leaves grow from base of plant and are roughly toothed. The whole plant exudes a milky juice when cut. Flowers February to November, but especially April and May. Largish golden-yellow flowers made up of numerous fine petals, on hollow stems up to 30 cm (1 ft) tall.

The dandelion is one of the most profuse of British weeds, and in late spring is liable to cover almost any grassy place with its blazing

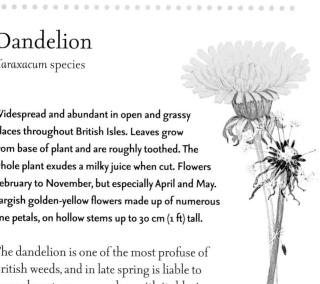

yellow flowers. Its leaves and consequently its roots can be found at almost any time of the year except the very coldest, which is welcome, given the wide range of food uses to which the plant can be put. But note the French name (pissenlit), and some of the English folk names (such as 'pissabed'), which should warn you that the plant has a reputation as a diuretic.

One use of the long white roots is to make a coffee substitute, which is remarkably like real coffee but is caffeine-free. Dig up the roots (from your own garden, or with the landowner's permission) in the autumn, when they are at their fattest and most mellow, and scrub well (though do not peel). Dry them thoroughly, preferably in the sun, and then roast in an oven until they are brittle. Grind them fairly coarsely and use as ordinary coffee.

Dandelion is especially useful as a salad plant, since the leaves can be gathered at almost any time of the year. Only after prolonged frost or snow is it impossible to find any. Choose the youngest leaves and strip them from the plant by hand. The root is quite strong enough to be unaffected by this sort of picking. If you have dandelions growing in your garden, try manuring them and covering the lower parts of the leaves with earth or a cardboard tube to blanch them like chicory. They did this in medieval gardens and produced gigantic plants as a result.

When you have sufficient leaves, trim off any excess stalk, and wash well. The roughly chopped leaves can be made into a good salad simply by dressing with olive oil, lemon juice and a trace of garlic. They can also be served in sandwiches with a dash of Worcester sauce, or tossed in fried bacon as pissenlit aux lardons.

The nineteenth-century French chef Marcel Boulestin recommended a salad made from equal quantities of dandelion 'hearts' (unopened flower-buds plus young surrounding leaves) and chopped beetroot.

Dandelion root, Japanese style

Chop the scrubbed roots into thin rings and sauté these
in vegetable oil, using about one tablespoonful of oil to
one cup of chopped roots. Then add a small amount of
water, a little salt, and cover the pan. Stew until the
roots are soft and most of the moisture and added
water have evaporated. Finally add a dash of soy sauce.

Tansy

Tanacetum vulgare

**Widespread in grassy and
rough ground throughout Europe.
Perennial, almost hairless, up
to 1.2 m (4 ft) high, with
toothed pinnate leaves and
yellow, button-like flowers in large clusters
from July to October.**

There was a time when tansy was one of the most widely
grown garden herbs. It was a key item in the housewife's
armoury of medicines, and had an extraordinarily wide
range of uses in the kitchen. All of which goes to show how
much our tastes have changed over the last few centuries, for
tansy is an unusually off-putting plant. It smells like a strong
chest ointment and has a hot, bitter taste. Used in excess it is
more than unpleasant, and can be a dangerous irritant to the
stomach.

Nevertheless, at Easter the young leaves were traditionally
served with fried eggs and used to flavour puddings made
from milk, flour and eggs. This may have been to symbolise
the bitter herbs eaten by the Jews at Passover, though one

sixteenth-century writer explained that it was to counteract the effects 'engendered of Fish in the Lent season'. He may have been on to something, as the quality of fish at that time no doubt encouraged the development of parasitic worms, and oil of tansy is quite effective as a vermifuge.

Earlier still, the juice was extracted from the chopped leaves and used to flavour omelettes. This gave the name *tansye* in the fifteenth century as a generic term for any herb-flavoured omelette. And there was a delightful medieval bubble-and-squeak, made from a fry-up of tansy leaves, green corn and violets, and served with orange and sugar.

Try the taste of tansy for yourself. Whatever you think of its flavour it is an attractive herb, with its clusters of golden, button-shaped flowers and ferny leaves.

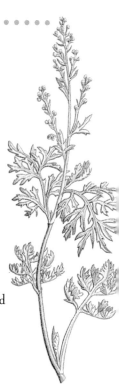

Wormwood

Artemisia absinthium

Frequent on rough ground, waste places and waysides in England and Wales. A strongly scented perennial, up to 1 m (3 ft), with yellowish flower-heads from July to August.

A bitter oil extracted from the flower-heads of this attractive silky-grey plant is the key ingredient of absinthe, that most potent of alcoholic drinks. The flowers have also been used in mainland Europe to counteract the greasiness of goose and duck dishes. Used in small quantities the herb has beneficial, tonic properties. But in excess it can be damaging to the heart. It also contains an anthelmintic called santonin, which is a hallucinogen if taken in overdose. Objects first appear blue and then change to yellow.

Mugwort
Artemisia vulgaris

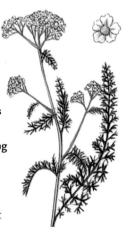

Common throughout lowland Britain, on waste ground and roadsides. A many-branched perennial, up to 1.5 m (5 ft). The flower-heads are reddish-brown and occur in clusters.

A common native relative of wormwood, whose bitter leaves have been used to flavour beer, and dried, as in tea.

Yarrow
Achillea millefolium

A sturdy, ferny perennial, 10–100 cm (4–40 inches) that grows in abundance in grassy places. Flowers consist of creamy-white disc florets and pink ray florets in flat-topped clusters, sometimes flowering right up to Christmas.

The Anglo-Saxons regarded yarrow as a powerful herb, providing protection against bad luck and illness. It also had a great reputation amongst herbalists as an astringent for wounds, although it was also believed to cause nosebleeds if one of the feathery leaves went up the nose.

Used in small quantities it can make a cool if rather bitter addition to salads. It can also be used as a cooked vegetable by removing the feathery leaves from the tough stems, boiling for five minutes, straining off the water, and then simmering in butter.

· ·

Common Chamomile
Chamaemelum nobile

Hairy, spreading perennial of grassy and heathy places. Flowers June to September.

Common chamomile is not common at all; in fact it is a rather rare plant largely confined to the south of England. It has a daisy-like flower and feathery leaves, but being a member of the huge and complex Asteraceae (Compositae) family this is scarcely enough to identify it. It can be told from the very similar scentless mayweed (Tripleurospermum inodorum) and corn chamomile (Anthemis arvensis) by an absence of down beneath its leaves. But its most conspicuous characteristic is its sweet apple scent, for which it was once much valued in rockeries, and even planted on lawns instead of grass. Indeed, the name is derived from an ancient Greek word meaning 'ground apple'.

Chamomile is still cultivated on a small scale for its flower-heads, which make a fine herbal tea. The heads are gathered when the petals just begin to turn down, and are used either fresh or dried. To dry the flowers, pick them carefully (using scissors) and spread on paper. Wait until the heads are papery and then store in a screw-top jar until needed.

- -

Oxeye Daisy
Leucanthemum vulgare

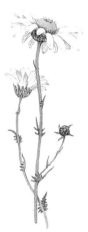

Widespread throughout the summer in grassy places, especially on rich soils. Erect stems, up to 75 cm (2–3 ft). One flower to each stem, each with a ring of white florets and a central yellow button.

John Evelyn reported that the roots of this, our commonest large daisy, were eaten as a salad vegetable in Spain.

- -

Lords-and-ladies, Arum Lily
Arum maculatum
☠ POISONOUS

A plant most country children are wisely taught to beware of. It grows abundantly in the shade of hedgerows and woods, like so many painted china ornaments. It is a plant which appears in several deceptively attractive disguises. The glossy, arrow-shaped leaves are amongst the very first foliage to appear in late winter. They are followed by a paler green cowl,

which encloses the club-shaped flower. In late summer the hood
withers and the flower produces a spike of shiny orange berries.

All stages and parts of the plant produce in the raw state an
acrid, burning juice, which is a serious irritant both
internally and externally. The root also contains this
poisonous element, yet if it is well baked it is completely
harmless. The cooked and ground roots were once in
demand in this country under the name Portland sago,
since the trade was centred round the Isle of Portland.
The powder was used like salep or as a substitute for
arrowroot.

Common Reed
Phragmites australis

**This is the common reed which so
readily forms dense beds in still, shallow
water. A very tall perennial, up to 3.5 m
(11–12 ft).**

When the stems of this familiar
waterside plant are punctured or
broken while still green they
slowly exude a sugary substance, which eventually hardens
into a gum. The North American Indians used to collect
this and break it into balls which they ate as sweets.
Another way of preparing a sweet from the plant was to cut
the reeds when still green, dry them, grind them and sift
out the flour. This contains so much sugar that when it is
placed near a fire it swells, browns, and can be eaten like
toasted marshmallow.

Spiked Star-of-Bethlehem, Bath Asparagus

Ornithogalum pyrenaicum

Very local and restricted. A hairless perennial, up to 80 cm (2–3 ft), with greyish linear leaves and tall spikes of flowers which are pale yellow on the inside and greenish-white on the outside, May to July.

An exquisite member of the lily family whose tall spikes of flowers are a distinctive feature of the limestone country around Bath and in the Avon valley in May and June. The young unopened flower spikes were gathered from the woods and hedgebanks and sold in the local markets for cooking like asparagus (a near relative). The species is too scarce to justify this kind of harvest in Britain today, though it is still used in France, and it remains one of the more historically interesting wild foods.

The spiked star-of-Bethlehem is strictly a Mediterranean native. Its distribution in Britain is concentrated around Wiltshire and Bath (though small colonies do occur elsewhere). It is a very common sight in this area, particularly near Bradford-on-Avon, and in spring can be almost as numerous as the bluebell. There has been some speculation that its abundance around Bath may be a legacy of the Roman occupation of the area, either accidentally or as a deliberate introduction.

Ramsons, Wild Garlic

Allium ursinum

Widespread and locally abundant in damp woods and hedgebanks throughout most of Europe. A bulbous perennial, up to 50 cm (20 inches). Leaves, broad and spear-like, often carpeting large areas. Flowers white, star-like, in a rounded umbel, April to June.

Large colonies of ramsons can often be smelt from some distance away, and garlic woods sometimes figured as landmarks in old land charters. But the taste of the leaf is milder than you might expect, and it makes an excellent substitute for garlic or spring onion in salads. One experimenter recommends the leaves added to peanut butter sandwiches.

For use in salads or sauces simply cut the leaves crosswise. Also try the leaves chopped in sour cream or mayonnaise. Or take advantage of their size and cut them into long, thin strips to lay crisscross over sliced tomatoes. They have an affinity with tomatoes, and one Italian chef in the Chilterns (who also makes flavoured olive oil by soaking ramsons leaves in it) sometimes adds them to tomato sauces instead of basil.

Several other species of the garlic and onion family can be used in the same way as ramsons, or as a coarse chives. These include three-cornered garlic (*Allium triquetrum*) quite commonly naturalised in the southwest, and wild onion or crow garlic (*Allium vineale*) common in arable fields and waysides.

Sand Leek

Allium scorodoprasum

This close relative of garlic – sometimes called 'rocambole' – grows very locally in hedgebanks and rough grass in northern England and southern Scotland. The plant has occasionally been taken into cultivation, or gathered in the wild state, and the bulbs and stems used in the same way as garlic.

Chives

Allium schoenoprasum

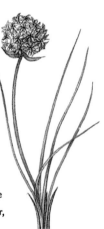

Chives is occasionally found in Britain as a naturalised escape, mainly on limestone cliffs near fresh water. It has long been cultivated as a herb, being especially prized by those who like the characteristic flavour of onions, but only in moderation. Its mildness and almost complete absence of a bulb have earned chives the name of 'infant onion'. It is a highly adaptable herb, going well with cream cheese, potatoes, cucumber, salads and omelettes.

Asparagus
Asparagus officinalis

A branched perennial reaching to 2 m (6 ft), with short, needle-like tufts of leaves, bell-shaped greenish-white flowers, May to August, and red berries from April to June.

There are two varieties of asparagus growing wild in Britain: wild asparagus (*Asparagus officinalis* ssp. *prostratus*), the prostrate, native subspecies; and garden asparagus (*A. o.* ssp. *officinalis*) an introduced variety that is naturalised in the wild and may appear on roadsides and waste ground almost anywhere.

Wild asparagus is particularly uncommon, now restricted to a few coastal localities in the southwest, and neither type grows as sumptuously as cultivated specimens, so picking is not recommended. The part of both plants which is eaten is the fat shoot, or 'spear', which grows from the rootstock in early summer.

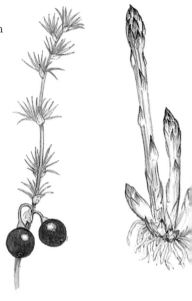

· ·

Early-purple Orchid

Orchis mascula

Widespread but local in woods, scrub and grassland. An erect perennial, 10–40 cm (4–16 inches). Leaves narrow, oblong and usually blotched purplish-black. Flowers purple, sometimes pink or white, April to June.

It would be irresponsible (and in most cases illegal) to dig up any of the dwindling colonies of early purple orchid, let alone for food. Yet this lilac-flowered woodland species has been one of the more fascinating and valuable of wild foods.

The tubers contain a starch-like polysaccharide called bassorine, and it is these tubers which have been used domestically, especially in the Middle East. In Turkey they are dug up after the plant has flowered, and made into a drink called *salep* or *sahlep*. The tubers are dried in the sun and ground into a rough flour, which is mixed with honey and cinnamon and stirred into hot milk until it thickens. The popularity of this drink – and of ice-cream flavoured with the *salep* flour – has resulted in a serious decline in orchid numbers in Turkey.

In Britain, an almost identical drink called saloop was a common soft drink long before the introduction of coffee houses. In Victorian books it is mentioned as a tea-break beverage of manual workers. Charles Lamb referred to a 'Salopian shop' in Fleet Street, and suggested that, at a cost of just three half-pence, a basin of saloop, accompanied by a slice of bread and butter (costing a halfpenny), made a good breakfast for a chimney-sweep. They made it with water more often than with milk, sometimes lacing it with spirits, sometimes brewing it so thick that it had to be eaten with a spoon.

Fungi

• •

Wild and exotic fungi are becoming increasingly prized and more commonly found on restaurant menus and on supermarket shelves, where their strange shapes and unusual textures often command a premium in terms of price.

Yet wild fungi remain the most misunderstood and maligned of all wild foods. There are 3,000 species of large-bodied fungi growing in the British Isles, though only twenty-odd of these are seriously poisonous. Admittedly, many hundreds of the remainder are inedible because of toughness, indigestibility or taste. But this scarcely seems sufficient to explain the blackening of the reputation of a whole biological category. Robert Graves suggested that our hostility towards fungi may be a hangover from the time when there were religious taboos against their use by any persons outside the priesthood. I would guess that there are more down-to-earth reasons than this. It would be foolish to pretend that the identification of fungi is as easy as the identification of flowering plants. They have fewer differentiating characteristics, and even within one species can vary enormously, in shape, size and colour. Even though the number of poisonous species is comparatively very small, each one resembles maybe half-a-dozen edible types.

The unearthly qualities of fungi no doubt exaggerate these worries. They rise up quickly, in lightless places. Many of them thrive on the dead or dying remains of other plants – or worse, of animals. Their shapes can bear resemblances to other organisms, to corals, brains, ears and sexual parts.

But there is no doubt that much of the discomfort we feel about fungi is conditioned by culture and fashion. We do, after all, consume vast quantities of cultivated mushrooms, and are increasingly happy to buy other species of fungi from shops. So the characteristic fungoid taste is not in itself repugnant. And in other parts of the world – in China, Russia, Scandinavia, Mediterranean Europe and Canada, for example – there is extensive use of wild fungi.

There are over a hundred quite edible species growing in this country, and it is sad that so many of them go to waste. They have no especial food value (though they contain more protein than vegetables and considerable quantities of vitamin D), but there are some intriguing tastes and textures, and they are worthwhile trying for these alone.

There are no general rules about when and where fungi may be found. They grow in all sorts of environments at all times of the year. But there are some guidelines which can be deduced from the way that they grow. Fungi are characterised by the fact that they do not contain any chlorophyll, and are thus unable to manufacture their own carbohydrates. They must live off those manufactured by other plants, either living or dead. Any ground which is rich in root structure or newly decaying plant litter is potentially good as a fungus bed. Mature woodlands and well-established pasture are both ideal environments. The more these host environments flourish, die and regenerate, the better off will be their attendant fungi. So although fungi have no use for direct light, they do prosper in areas where the underground growth and cycling of their hosts is stimulated by light: hedges, woodland clearings and paths, etc. They also like warmth and damp, and a year which begins with a long, fine summer, and continues with a wet, mild autumn, is likely to be as good for fungi as it is for other types of fruit. It is the right balance of sunlight, moisture and warmth which seems to be crucial. In wet summers fungi tend to appear more in woodland clearings; in dry summers in the shady, moisture-retaining spots.

Some fungi appear in the spring and others can live through the winter. But the greatest number appear in the late summer and disappear with the first hard frosts.

Some picking rules

The following are a few suggestions about picking and preparation which apply to all fungi, and which will help guarantee you have good specimens this season, and more to come back to next.

1 Only pick those which satisfy all the criteria on size, colour, time of year and environment that are given on the following pages. These have been chosen so that it is very difficult to make a mistake if you follow them to the letter. There are several other published guides which can help you make an accurate identification. If you are in any doubt about the identification, do not eat it.

2 Do not pick specimens which are so old that they have started to decay, or so young that they have not yet developed their identifying characteristics.

3 Avoid gathering on very wet days. Many fungi are highly porous, and a blewit, for instance, can soak up its own weight of water in a few hours. Moisture not only spoils the taste and texture but creates conditions where decomposition can proceed more quickly.

4 When picking fungi, do not cut them with a knife, or yank them out of the ground, either. You will need the whole stalk (stipe), and any sheath (volva) for a full identification. The fungi we pick are simply the fruit bodies of the fungus proper, which is a complex net of fine threads called the mycelium growing underground. If this is broken by too careless picking, the fungus can be damaged. The best way of picking a fungus is to twist it gently until it breaks free.

5 It is best to cut the earthy part of the stipe away before putting the mushroom into a basket. This will prevent it soiling those mushrooms already gathered, and will give a fair idea whether any maggots or insects have got into the cap via the stem.

6 Gather your crop into an open, well-ventilated basket, not your pockets or a polythene bag. Fungi decay very quickly, and heat, congestion and stale air accelerate this process.

7 Go through all your specimens again carefully before cooking. Check their identification and discard any you are not confident about. Indigestion brought on by uncertainty about whether you have done yourself in can be just as uncomfortable as real food poisoning. Remember there are no infallible tricks with sixpences or salt which can identify all poisonous species.

8 To be especially careful cut each fungus in half and throw away any that are maggot-ridden or possessed of suspicious white gills (most of the deadly *Amanita* species have these). Also cut away decaying or wet pieces.

9 Clean the fungi before cooking, by brushing or cutting away dirt. There is no need to wash them or peel them, unless it is specifically stated in the text. Use them within 24 hours of picking.

10 In common with other new foods it is as well to try a fairly small portion the first time you eat any species. It is just possible that it may 'disagree with you'.

Having prepared your fungi, remember that there are many other ways of using them beyond the recipes given here for individual species.

Drying is a useful way of preserving them for the winter. Special drying trays and small ovens are now available commercially, but to dry the fungi more cheaply, simply cut prepared specimens into slices about 2 mm thick and keep in a warm place or a dry current of air. Threading the slices (or the whole caps of smaller specimens) onto a string is a convenient and attractive way of doing this. They are dry when they feel crisp to the fingers and can be easily crumbled into small pieces. The fungi can be reconstituted by boiling in water for about twenty minutes.

Fungi can also be pickled by being simmered in water for about ten minutes, drained and put in jars under ordinary pickling vinegar.

All edible fungi can be made into soup, using the recipe on p. 212, or ketchup (p. 218). There is also scope for a whole new range of recipes based on a view of them as fruits rather than savouries. Try them stewed with sugar, like plums, or added to cakes and puddings, as if they were currants.

Finally, find out if your local natural history society or wildlife trust holds fungus forays in the autumn. These traditional foraging expeditions have been revived all over the country, and there is no better way of getting to know the situations in which the different species grow, and how to look out for their identifying characteristics.

Morel

Morchella esculenta

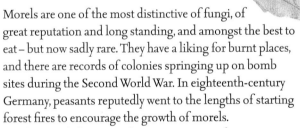

Woodland clearings, old orchards and pastures (especially sandy soils), under broad-leaved trees, especially ash and elm. Unusual in appearing in spring, from March to May. The cap is wrinkled like a coarse sponge, variable in shape and colour but usually 3–6 cm (1–2 inches) across, light or dark brown. Cap fused to stem, which is white and hollow with no ring.

Morels are one of the most distinctive of fungi, of great reputation and long standing, and amongst the best to eat – but now sadly rare. They have a liking for burnt places, and there are records of colonies springing up on bomb sites during the Second World War. In eighteenth-century Germany, peasants reputedly went to the lengths of starting forest fires to encourage the growth of morels.

The morel's honeycomb structure means that it is apt to collect dirt and insects, and the caps must be cut in half and rinsed under running water – or dusted with a paintbrush – before use. They are sometimes blanched in boiling water before cooking.

Morels make good additions to stews and soups, and, being hollow, can be stuffed and baked. Sliced horizontally they produce crinkle-edged golden rings that can ornament omelettes or mushroom soups.

Morels only appear for a few days each spring, often after warm rains, and if you are lucky enough to find a hoard it is worth preserving them. They freeze well, in airtight plastic

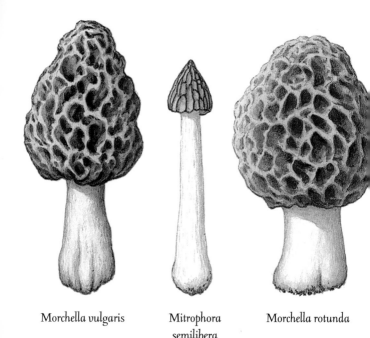

Morchella vulgaris   Mitrophora   Morchella rotunda
                   semilibera

bags, or can be dried. Cut them in half vertically and hang up in a warm room until they are crisp.

Carter's eighteenth-century *Herbal* gives a recipe for 'fricassy of morelles' – unusual for a time when fungi were generally regarded with suspicion:

'Cleanse them from the Sand by washing them, and brown a Piece of Butter gold colour, and toss them up, and their own Liquor will stove them; season them only with Pepper, Salt, and Nutmeg, and an Onion, and a little minc'd Parsley; when stov'd tender, toss them up as a Fricassy, with the Yolk of an Egg and a little White Wine, and a little Cream and thick Butter, and so serve them; and you may garnish with Lemon.'

The following morels are also edible and good:

Morchella vulgaris

As *M. esculenta* but with more sinuous and complex pitting.

Mitrophora semilibera

Quite common in damp copses on heavy soil in spring. Cap 2–4 cm (³/₄–1¹/₂ inches), olive-brown, slightly pitted with rather regular vertical ribs. Stipe creamy-white, hollow.

Morchella rotunda

In woods on heavy soils. Late spring. Cap 10–20 cm (4–8 inches), yellowish brown. Stipe rather stocky.

· ·

False Morel

Gyromitra esculenta

☠ POISONOUS

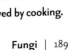

The only species that might conceivably be mistaken for morels. Rather scarce, found under pines on sandy soils, and near the sites of bonfires in spring, like morel, but only really common in the central Highlands. Cap 5–10 cm (2–4 inches), with brain-like lobes, russet to rusty brown in colour. Flesh pale, bitter, strong-smelling. Stem short, stout, hollow, multi-chambered like the cap (the true morel has a single-chambered stem). The false morel is highly poisonous when raw, but the toxins are destroyed by cooking.

Truffle
Tuber aestivum

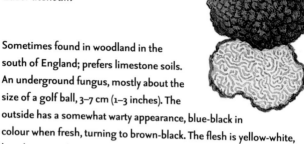

Sometimes found in woodland in the south of England; prefers limestone soils. An underground fungus, mostly about the size of a golf ball, 3–7 cm (1–3 inches). The outside has a somewhat warty appearance, blue-black in colour when fresh, turning to brown-black. The flesh is yellow-white, later brown with white marbling.

The highly prized Périgord or black truffle (Tuber melanosporum) is not found in Britain, though the summer truffle (T. aestivum) does occur. Truffles are all but impossible to find without specially trained animals. Truffle hunting is still part of the rural economy of mainland Europe, particularly in France and Italy, and there was once a lively traffic in them in some of the southern counties of England, where they were sniffed out of beech woods by Spanish poodles.

The last professional truffle hunter in Britain, Alfred Collins, retired in 1930. Before that time truffle hunting in the Winterslow area of Wiltshire had a tradition going back 300 years. Between November and March Alfred would scour the countryside together with his dogs. Dogs have to be trained to dig out truffles, in the same way that they are trained to sniff out drugs by police and customs officers, but pigs (which were not much used in Britain) hunt for truffles naturally. Apparently Alfred Collins became so experienced in his trade that he could smell truffles while they were still in the ground. He could also feel them underfoot, and judge from clouds of flies whether a truffle was lying beneath the topsoil.

It was clearly a thriving small business, providing income for all sorts of people. In a 1971 article for Country Life, J. E. Manners described how the truffles were found and distributed:

'Normally, the hunter worked up wind and his dogs could scent the truffles frequently from a distance of twenty yards upwards. Truffles were invariably sold to private customers so they rarely came on the market. They only kept for about four days before losing flavour so they were always posted off as soon as possible in cardboard shoe boxes, which the children collected from the bootmaker for a penny each. Any not despatched were eaten by children on bread and butter. They could be preserved in vinegar. Like mushrooms they grew and then dispersed fairly quickly, the process taking about two days.'

Although the milder flavour of the summer truffle is inferior to that of its Périgord counterpart, it should certainly be regarded as an exciting find. Gently brush any soil away from the skin, and make sure you slice it thinly to get maximum use out of it! It can be added to stuffings and patés, and can make luxurious omelettes and scrambled eggs. The truffle can also be used to flavour oil, which also serves to preserve the fungus, though it will reduce its flavour. Truffle oil is very rich and should be used sparingly.

Truffle soufflé omelette
(from Rose Elliot)

A sumptuous cross between a soufflé and an omelette is created by folding beaten egg whites into egg yolks that have been mixed well with a little water and seasoning. Pour the mixture into a heated and buttered pan and cook until golden underneath. Put the pan under the grill until the top is golden, then make a cut across the middle of the omelette (but not right through), sprinkle truffle shavings over one half, and fold the other half over. Serve with a little parsley sprinkled on top.

Tuber aestivum can be confused with the false truffle, or hart's truffle (*Elaphomyces granulatus*). This is one of the most frequently found underground fungi, developing just below the surface in woodland soil, especially in coniferous woods with pine. About the size of a large marble – the ones that used to be so highly prized in school playgrounds – the false truffle's skin is thick, warty and red-brown. The flesh is flecked purple-brown and darkens as the spores mature. This species is not edible, and when uncovered can be told by the fact that it has no distinctive smell.

Cauliflower Fungus, Sparassis

Sparassis crispa

Found at the base of pine stumps or living trees, August to November. Resembles a large

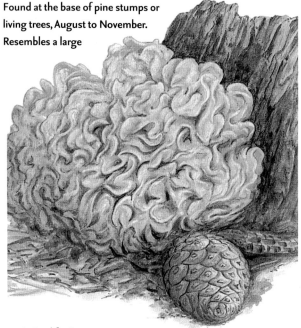

round natural sponge or the heart of a cauliflower, 15–40 cm (6–15 inches) across, with *flat*, twisted and very divided branches. The colour varies with age from pale cream to ochre.

If you are lucky enough to find a *Sparassis* nestling at the bottom of a pine (the Swiss call it 'the broody hen') it should be cut off from its thick fleshy stalk with a knife. Only young specimens should be gathered, as the old ones are tough and bitter.

Cut the *Sparassis* into sections, making it easier to clean, and remove any brown or spongy parts. Then wash thoroughly to remove any dirt and insects from the folds. An old recipe for very young specimens is to bake them in a casserole with butter, parsley, a little garlic, and some stock and seasoning. They taste mild and pleasantly nutty, which also makes them a good addition to soups and stews. Rather older specimens are best dried until they are brittle, for future use as flavouring.

- -

Ramaria formosa
☠ POISONOUS

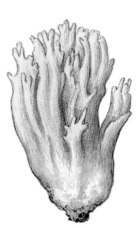

Uncommon, under broadleaved trees. Pink, coral-like branches up to about 15 cm (6 inches) tall. This is the only slightly dangerous species with which *Sparassis* could conceivably be confused. It has pink, rounded branches. *Ramaria formosa* is purgative, but not seriously poisonous.

Horn of Plenty
Craterellus cornucopoides

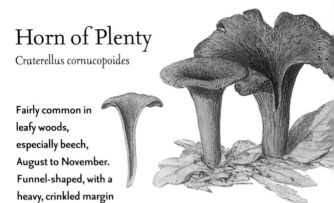

**Fairly common in
leafy woods,
especially beech,
August to November.
Funnel-shaped, with a
heavy, crinkled margin
to the cap, 2–8 cm (1–3 inches) across, browny-black in colour.
Lower surface of cap continuous with stem, and smooth or slightly
wrinkled. No ring.**

The flesh of this species is thin and leathery and tastes of
earth when eaten raw, but it is highly prized for culinary
purposes. When you get it home, check that the base is free
from dirt and insects before sautéing until softened. The
caps can then be stuffed, or used in sauces or soups. Horn of
plenty is also good for drying.

• •

Chanterelle
Cantharellus cibarius

**Fairly common in all kinds of woodland, but especially beech,
between July and December. Shaped like a funnel, 2–7 cm (1–3
inches) across. Egg-yolk yellow in colour and smelling slightly of
apricots. Gills like fan-vaulting or veins, shallow, much forked and
continuous with the stem. No ring.**

Chanterelles have long been regarded as among the most
desirable fungi. An eighteenth-century writer even said that

if they were placed in the mouths of dead men they would come to life again. In her book Food in England, Dorothy Hartley wrote

'You find them, suddenly, in the autumn woods, sometimes clustered so close that they look like a torn golden shawl dropped amongst the dead leaves and sticks.'

Because they are seldom attacked by insects, and are unlikely to be confused with any dangerous species, chanterelles (girolles) are extensively eaten throughout mainland Europe. They are slightly tougher than some other fungi and should be stewed slowly in milk for at least ten minutes. The result is delicately perfumed and slightly peppery. They can also be sliced and fried with garlic, parsley or lemon juice. Perhaps because of colour sympathy, chanterelles have always been associated with eggs, and there is scarcely any better way of serving previously cooked specimens than in omelettes or with scrambled eggs.

Be careful of false chanterelle (Hygrophoropsis aurantiaca) which is not worth eating and may be poisonous to some. This species is more common with conifers and on heathland. It is more orange than the true chanterelle, and lacks the fruity smell. Also avoid jack o'lantern (Omphalotus olearius) which occasionally appears on sweet chestnut and oak trees in southern England. It has an unpleasant smell. Finally there are two Cortinarius species (C. orellanus and C. speciosissimus), which are both rare but poisonous.

Cantharellus infundibuliformis

Found in clusters in all kinds of woodland, July to January. Funnel-shaped, with a slightly crinkled margin. Cap 2.5–5 cm (1–2 inches) across and dark brown. Stem deep yellow. Gills fold-like and branched as in the chanterelle. No ring.

This fairly common relative of the chanterelle can be used in much the same way.

. . . .

Wood Hedgehog
Hydnum repandum

Uncommon in all kinds of woodland, August to November. The cap is irregularly shaped, up to 15 cm (6 inches) across, and is covered with a matt buffish to pink skin, smooth and often cracked, like fine leather. The 'gills' take the form of unmistakable tiny white spines of unequal length. Stem short, stout, whitish. No ring.

The genus *Hydnum* is unique amongst fungi in having spines instead of gills, and all the commoner species having this characteristic are edible. Once you have picked the fungi, any dirt trapped in the spines can be removed with a knife. It is best to remove the spines completely from older caps.

The wood hedgehog is the commonest *Hydnum* species, and is good to eat once its slightly bitter taste has been removed. This is best done by boiling the chopped fungus

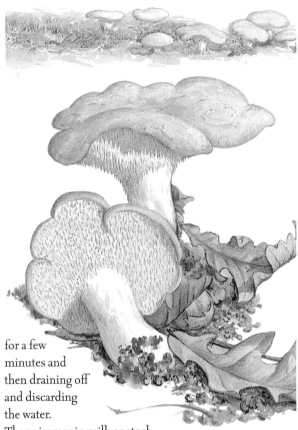

for a few
minutes and
then draining off
and discarding
the water.
Then simmer in milk or stock
for a further ten minutes, or slice and
fry lightly. Serve on toast with a dash of sherry sprinkled
over the top. Its firm texture makes it good for freezing
(once cooked), and it can also be pickled.

Sarcodon imbricatum

Occurs occasionally in sandy conifer woods between August and
November, particularly in hilly districts. A conventional mushroom-

shaped cap fungus, greyish brown in colour, with a scaly cap and the usual spiny gill structure of the Hydnum family.

This close relative of the wood hedgehog has an excellently strong, spicy flavour, and is consequently useful as a flavouring.

Beefsteak Fungus

Fistulina hepatica

Occurs on living trees, especially old oak or sweet chestnut, August to October. A large, red bracket fungus, 20–40 cm (8–16 inches) in diameter. Resembles an ox tongue, rough and sticky, becoming drier and smoother with age. The top is reddish brown, and the underside is covered with minute yellow pores which exude a blood-like juice when bruised.

This is an aptly named fungus, for the flesh when cut looks and feels like prime raw beef. Regrettably, the beefsteak fungus does not really fulfil its visual promise, and the meat is rather tough and bitter. It is best chopped small and fried well with some other fairly strongly flavoured ingredients, such as onions and herbs. Stewing repeatedly in water, changing the water each time, can remove the acid that makes the fungus bitter. Even then the acrid taste is not completely destroyed, though in good specimens it is not unpleasantly reminiscent of unripe tomatoes.

St George's Mushroom

Calocybe gambosa

Old grassland, downs and dunes throughout Britain, April to June. Cap 5–12 cm (2–5 inches) across when young, later flatter with wavy edges. Cap, gills and stem all creamy-white in colour.

This is the French *mousseron*, unmistakable as the only large white mushroom to appear in spring – traditionally around St George's Day, 23 April. It likes old grassland – chalk downland, grassy woodland edges and even churchyards. It has a strong, mealy, almost yeasty smell, though this is less pronounced in younger specimens.

St George's mushrooms are firm, not often attacked by insects, and can generally be treated like field mushrooms. But some people find the aroma of mature specimens a little too heady and rich, and they are probably best used in dishes where there is another strongly flavoured ingredient – for instance in quiches with cheese and spinach or spring greens.

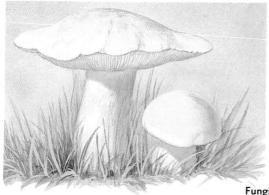

Field Blewit

Lepista saeva

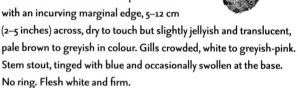

**Not uncommon in grassy pastures,
October to December. The cap is flattish
with an incurving marginal edge, 5–12 cm
(2–5 inches) across, dry to touch but slightly jellyish and translucent,
pale brown to greyish in colour. Gills crowded, white to greyish-pink.
Stem stout, tinged with blue and occasionally swollen at the base.
No ring. Flesh white and firm.**

Blewits, named after the bluish-violet tinge of their stems,
were one of the few fungi once sold commercially in Britain.
The trade was especially strong in the Midlands, and it is
from there that the traditional way of cooking blewits as
tripe comes.

Blewits often grow in large rings, and it is easy to
overlook them in the late autumn, for their flat irregular
caps look like dead leaves scattered over the field. Pick them
on a dry day (they are very porous), clean, and chop off their
stems. One way to serve this excellent fungus is to cook
them like tripe (see below) – which is probably not entirely
fortuitous, for their aromatic taste and jellyish texture are
indeed reminiscent of tripe. Fried with onions, and perhaps
chopped potato, they also make an excellent omelette filling.
Or they can be dried, pickled or frozen.

Blewits, tripe-style

Remove the stems and chop them finely with an
equal amount of onions, then pack this mixture
round the caps with a little chopped sage and bacon
fat. Just cover the blewits with milk and simmer for
half an hour. Pour off the liquid, thicken with flour
and butter and seasoning and pour back over the

fungi mixture. Simmer for another quarter of an
hour, and then serve the whole mixture inside a ring
of mashed potatoes, with toast and apple sauce.

Wood Blewit

Lepista nuda

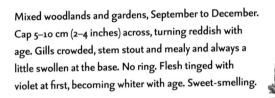

**Mixed woodlands and gardens, September to December.
Cap 5–10 cm (2–4 inches) across, turning reddish with
age. Gills crowded, stem stout and mealy and always a
little swollen at the base. No ring. Flesh tinged with
violet at first, becoming whiter with age. Sweet-smelling.**

The woodland equivalent of the field blewit, very similar but
bluish or violet all over when young. Use as field blewits, but
do not eat raw, as they can be indigestible.

Honey Fungus

Armillaria mellea

**Abundant throughout Britain on tree stumps, roots, buried
branches, September to December. Tufts of caps 5–12 cm (2–5 inches)
across, yellow to olive-brown, convex with brownish scales when
young, flattening with age. Gills creamy-white, darkening with age.
Stipe yellowish, with a shaggy yellow ring.**

Honey fungus is a destructive parasite on all kinds of
timber, recognisable from the black rhizomes encircling its
host, which resemble a network of leather bootlaces.

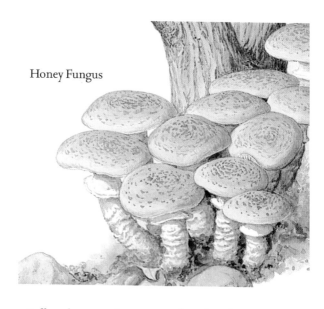

Honey Fungus

Collect the caps when young, when the gills are white, and do not eat raw. Blanch before cooking, then fry slowly. They have a strong flavour and firm texture, and are best served in small quantities on the first tasting, as they can be quite rich for some people. Probably best added to stews.

Anise Cap

Clitocybe odora

A small fungus which occurs in the litter of mixed woodlands, especially beech and oak on chalky soils, August to November. The whole fungus is a uniform blue-green colour, and has a strong, unmistakable smell of aniseed. Cap 3–6 cm (1–2 inches) across, becoming lighter, flatter and wavy with age.

The aniseed smell persists on drying, and either fresh or dried the anise cap can be used as a flavouring. It is good for flavouring fish in place of fennel.

Velvet Shank, Winter Mushroom

Flammulina velutipes

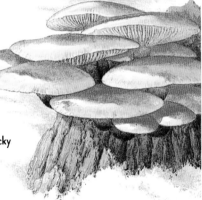

Common in clusters on stumps and trunks between September and March. The caps are thin, about 2–8 cm (1–3 inches) across, sticky and glistening, and honey-yellow to orange-red in colour. Gills broad and pale yellow. Stem thin, tough, often curved, dark brown in colour and covered with a dark velvety down. The flesh is thin, whitish and rubbery with no smell.

This is one of the few fungi able to survive through frosts. During the winter months there is consequently very little chance that it might be confused with another species. They can even be picked while frozen, and either stored in a deep-freeze or added to stews and casseroles. Make sure you discard the stems and wipe the stickiness off the cap before using them. Add a few towards the last stages of cooking a stew and they will float on the surface like fungal water-lilies. The Japanese *enoki*, or *enokitake*, is a cultivated variety of this species.

Fairy-ring Champignon

Marasmius oreades

Very common on lawns and short grassland, April to December, often growing in 'fairy rings'. The cap, 2–5 cm (1–2 inches) across, has a slight bump in the centre. When moist, the top is smooth and buffish in colour, and when dry, the skin wrinkles, becomes hard and leathery and changes to pale tan in colour. Gills wide and usually free of the stipe, which is tough and fibrous. The smell is pleasantly aromatic, a little like new-mown hay scented with bitter almonds.

This is one of the best and most versatile toadstools – though care must be taken to distinguish it from somewhat similar small, white and poisonous *Clitocybe* species that can grow on lawns.

The fairy-ring champignon's natural tendency to dry out is one of its great virtues, and means that the caps can be easily preserved by threading them on strings and hanging them for a week or two in a dry, well-ventilated room. Discard the tough stems before threading. They can be reconstituted by soaking in water overnight.

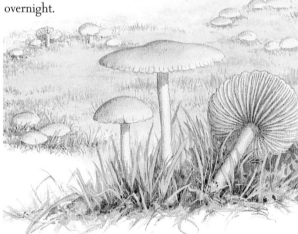

The other virtues of the fairy-ring champignon are its almond fragrance and nutty texture – it is prized for its flavour rather than its bulk. Add them to stews and casseroles, or fry them with chopped almonds or hazelnuts.

Oyster Mushroom

Pleurotus ostreatus

Common on dead or dying branches of beech and ash round the year, though principally in late autumn and winter. This is a bracket fungus, growing on the branch or trunk in shelves up to 20 cm (8 inches) across. The cap is shell-shaped, convex at first, then flat, grey or slate-blue in colour. Gills white and deep. Flesh white, soft, rubbery.

The oyster mushroom tends to be rather tough, and you should choose young specimens and cook them thoroughly. But when you find it, it is usually possible to gather considerable quantities from the clusters in which it invariably grows, so it should not be passed over. Inspect carefully for maggots when cleaning. Because of their comparatively mild flavour, oyster mushrooms can be served with fairly rich sauces. They can also be grilled, added to stews and casseroles, and dried.

Oyster mushrooms are one of the few wild species that are now being successfully cultivated. Many supermarkets stock them, and it is possible to grow your own from specially prepared and prespawned 'logs'.

Deep-fried oyster mushrooms

Slice the mushrooms into pieces not more than 1 cm
(½ inch) thick, sprinkling with a few drops of lemon
juice, turning in seasoned flour, then in beaten egg and
finally in breadcrumbs. The slices should then be fried in
deep oil until golden.

Oyster mushrooms in Madeira sauce

Slice the mushrooms about 1 cm (½ inch) thick, and
fry in oil for 5 minutes until the juices begin to flow.
Sprinkle a little flour into the pan, and then stir in a
glass of Madeira or sherry. Add a beaten egg yolk and
seasoning. Simmer and stir until the mixture
thickens. Serve on toast or fried bread.

- -

Amanita species

The Amanita family contains some of the commonest and
most toxic of all poisonous fungi. All the dangerous species
have a white sheath surrounding the base of the stem, a white
ring, and white gills. Avoid all fungi that have this combination.

Panthercap

Amanita pantherina

☠ POISONOUS

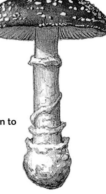

Rather uncommon under broadleaved
trees. Cap 5–10 cm (2–4 inches) across, fawn to
russet-brown in colour, flecked with pure
white scales. Gills, stem, ring and sheath
white.

Deathcap

Amanita phalloides

☠ DEADLY POISONOUS

Quite common under
broadleaved trees, and
occasionally conifers.
Cap 5–12 cm (2–5 inches) across,
smooth, yellowish green. Gills,
stem and ring white. Sheath
very pronounced, like an open sack.

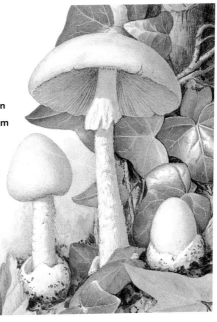

Destroying Angel

Amanita virosa

☠ DEADLY POISONOUS

Uncommon under
broadleaved trees on
acid soils. Cap 5–8 cm
(2–3 inches) across.
All parts – cap, gills,
stem, ring, sheath –
pure white.

Fly Agaric

Amanita muscaria

☠ POISONOUS

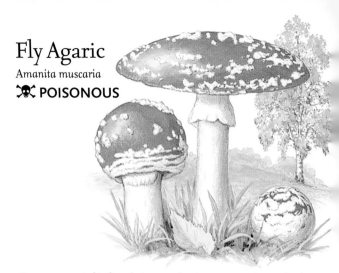

Very common in birch and pine woods. Cap 10–20 cm (4–8 inches) across, bright vermilion fading to orange, and usually flecked with white scales. Gills and stem white. Ring white, with remnants of veil. Sheath white.

- -

Parasol Mushroom

Macrolepiota procera

Wood margins, grassy clearings, roadsides, July to November. A large fungus, up to 30 cm (12 inches) tall and 20 cm (8 inches) across. When young the cap resembles an old-fashioned, domed beehive. It then spreads out flat but always retains its dark central prominence. It is dry, scaly, brown to grey-brown. Gills white and detached from the stem. Stem tall, slender, hollow and bulbous at the base and slightly scaly like the cap. Large white double ring which eventually becomes completely free of the stem so that it can be moved up and down.

With its large, dry cap, the parasol is one of the best of our edible fungi. It is also one of the most distinctive, and can often be seen from afar because of its size and preference for open spaces. The parasol rises closed, held to the stem by its large white ring. It then breaks free and opens like an umbrella. For the best combination of size and tenderness it should be picked just when the cap begins to open.

To cook, remove the stems and fry the caps quickly in oil or butter like field mushrooms. Alternatively, to avoid the caps soaking up too much fat, coat them first in batter or breadcrumbs. The shape of the more mature caps makes them suitable for making into fritters. Prepare the caps by removing the stalks, and wiping clean. Then dip them, whole, into flour, then batter, and deep-fry in oil for about five minutes.

Stuffed parasols

Because of their shape young parasols are ideal for stuffing. Choose specimens that are still cup-shaped, cut off and discard the stems and fill with a sage and onion stuffing (or with mince or sausage meat if you want a more substantial dish). Arrange them their natural way up in a baking tray. For even more flavour, fasten a small strip of bacon fat to the top of each parasol with a skewer. Cook in the oven for about 30 minutes, basting once or twice.

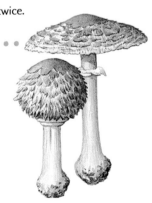

Shaggy Parasol
Macrolepiota rhacodes

Not uncommon on rich ground, though prefers more shade than the common parasol. July to November. Very similar to

previous species, but the cap is scalier and the stem quite smooth. Flesh white but reddens on cutting.

A lookalike species which can be cooked in the same way as the common parasol. Note that the shaggy parasol has rarely caused digestive upsets and rashes on skin.

● ●

Field Mushroom

Agaricus campestris

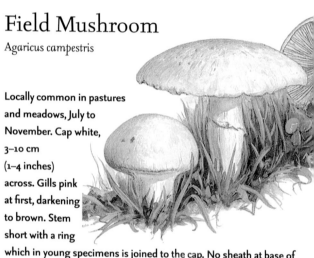

Locally common in pastures and meadows, July to November. Cap white, 3–10 cm (1–4 inches) across. Gills pink at first, darkening to brown. Stem short with a ring which in young specimens is joined to the cap. No sheath at base of stem, and no unpleasant smell.

Field mushrooms have a special liking for meadows manured by horses, and the passing of horse-drawn transport, followed by increasing intensification of agriculture and the use of artificial fertilisers, has seriously affected the abundance of mushroom fields. There was a time when such fields might experience a 'white-out', when the precisely right combination of temperature, humidity and soil condition produced so many mushrooms simultaneously that the field appeared to have been covered overnight by snow. But in normal quantities they are, paradoxically, one of the less easy fungi to identify exactly. There is virtually nothing which could be mistaken for a sparassis or a chanterelle, but there are one or two white-capped meadow fungi which can be taken for mushrooms by the careless. But if you study cultivated mushrooms carefully, and go only for similar pink-gilled, sheathless specimens from the wild, you are unlikely to make a mistake.

Gathering mushrooms is a skill which has to be learned. They do not loom up above the grass as in fairy-story illustrations. In the rather dense pasture that is their natural habitat they are sometimes only visible as bright white patches in the grass when you are almost on top of them. You must train your eyes to scan no more then a few feet in front of you as you methodically quarter a field. When you find one, examine the area around it especially thoroughly, as mushrooms, like other fungi, tend to grow in colonies from the parent mycelium.

When you have your mushrooms check them again to make sure there are none with greenish-tinged or warty caps, or with remnants of sheath at the bottom of the stems. And until you are expert at recognising the 'jizz' of mushrooms it is as well to be doubly cautious and cut each specimen in half vertically. Discard any with pure white gills, or that quickly stain pink or yellow. The blusher (Amanita rubescens) and the yellow-staining mushroom (Agaricus xanthodermus) can both be mistaken for the field mushroom, and though neither of them is dangerously poisonous, they can cause digestive disturbances.

There is no need to peel mushrooms – indeed the taste will be diminished if you do. Simply wipe the caps with a dampish cloth and cut off the base of the stem. The very best way of cooking mushrooms is to fry them in bacon fat as soon as possible after collecting. The secret is to give them no more than three or four minutes in the pan. Field mushrooms tend to contain more water than cultivated, and if they are cooked for too long, they stew in their own liquid and become limp and mushy. Making soup from your wild mushrooms avoids this danger. Young field mushrooms can also be used raw in salads, and ripe, dark-gilled ones for ketchup (see recipe on p. 218).

Mushroom soup
Simmer the chopped caps and stems in seasoned milk for about 30 minutes with no other ingredients at all. Liquidise in a blender if desired. The result is a smooth, light soup which is good hot or cold.

Mushroom pâté
200 g (8 oz) field mushrooms
1 onion
1 tomato
1 rasher of bacon (optional)
1 egg, beaten
Seasoning to taste

1 Chop the mushrooms with the onion, tomato and bacon. Cook slowly in a little oil until the mushrooms begin to sweat, and simmer for 10 minutes. If they give off a great deal of liquid, drain some of this away.
2 Cool and transfer to a blender and blitz until the mixture is smooth.
3 Return to the pan, add seasoning and herbs to taste, perhaps a pinch of chilli powder, and finally the beaten egg. Stir over a low heat until the texture thickens.
4 Refrigerate for at least 12 hours, when it will acquire the consistency of a pâté, and a surprisingly meaty taste.

The following relatives of the field mushroom can all be treated in similar ways, and are all edible and good:

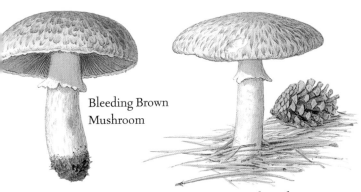

Bleeding Brown Mushroom

Brown Wood Mushroom

Bleeding Brown Mushroom

Agaricus haemorrhoidarius

Common under broadleaved trees, especially oak, among soil and dead leaves. Cap 10–12 cm (4–5 inches), hazel-brown with faint reddish-brown scales. Gills pink. Flesh white, turning blood-red when cut. Double ring. September.

Brown Wood Mushroom

Agaricus silvaticus

Common under conifers. Cap 5–9 cm (2–3¹/₂ inches), covered with russet-brown scales. Gills reddish. Flesh white, staining orange-red, then blood-red, when cut. Large ring. August to October.

Wood Mushroom

Agaricus silvicola

Occasional in deciduous and coniferous woodland. Cap 5–10 cm (2–4 inches), white, turning yellow and eventually orange. Gills pinkish-grey. Flesh white, becoming yellow. Smells of aniseed. August to November.

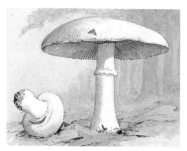

Wood Mushroom

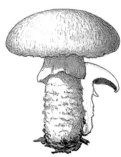

Agaricus macrosporus

Agaricus macrosporus

The usual Agaricus of pastures in the Highlands. Cap 20–30 cm (8–12 inches), very fleshy and silky-white, remains convex. Flesh thick, white, flushing pink at the base, smelling slightly of aniseed.

Agaricus augustus

Occasional in parks, gardens and broadleaved woods. Cap 12–18 cm (5–7 inches), covered with golden-brown scales. Flesh white, flushing pink towards the base and yellowing in the cap. Smells of bitter almonds.

Cultivated Mushroom
Agaricus bisporus

Occasional in fields and gardens, and on manure. Cap 5–10 cm (2–4 inches), white, browning slightly on the top. Flesh grows slightly pink with age and reddens when cut. Large ring. This is the most common species in cultivation.

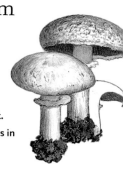

Agaricus bitorquis

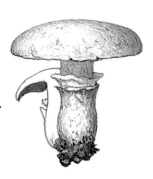

Common in southeast England on waste ground, field edges, pavement cracks, etc. Cap 6–12 cm (2^1/$_2$–5 inches), white. Flesh dingy white, turning pale wine-coloured eventually. Smells of almonds.

Horse Mushroom

Agaricus arvensis

Very like a large field mushroom. Grows in similar habitats and at the same time of year. Can be up to 30 cm (1 ft) across when mature. Cap white, yellowing with age. Bruises yellow-brown on handling. Gills greyer than in the field mushroom. Smells pleasantly of almonds.

This close cousin of the field mushroom is also becoming uncommon. But it is a large, meaty and flavourful fungus, and if you only succeed in finding one mature specimen you have enough for a good meal. Remember to check for maggots. Avoid specimens that bruise bright yellow, in case they are the poisonous yellow-staining mushroom.

If horse mushrooms are still dome-shaped they can be stuffed with tomatoes. If they are flat, grill them whole like steaks. Otherwise use as field mushroom.

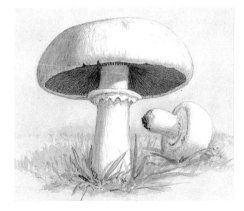

Horse mushroom and red currants

Stew the mushrooms in milk, drain, set in a dish of white sauce, and then garnish with whole red currants made hot to the point of bursting. The dish is a contrast in colour and texture: the bright and sharp against the dark and fleshy.

Yellow-staining Mushroom

Agaricus xanthodermus

☠ POISONOUS

Parks, open woodland and gardens under broadleaved trees. Very similar in appearance to a small horse mushroom. Cap 5–11 cm (2–4 inches) across, creamy-white, often with small brown scales in the middle. Gills white at first, turning grey-pink and finally dark brown. Stipe turns bright chrome-yellow if cut near the base. The smell is also distinctive, reminiscent of ink or iodine. Can cause acute, if temporary, digestive upsets in susceptible persons.

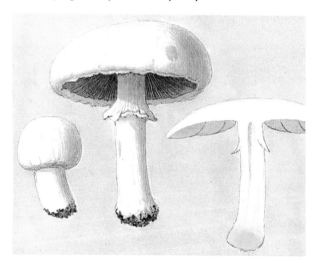

Agaricus placomyces
☠ POISONOUS

Similar to the yellow-stainer except
that the cap is covered with dark
scales. Indigestible rather than
poisonous, but best avoided.

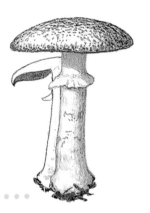

Shaggy Inkcap, Lawyer's Wig

Coprinus comatus

Fields, road verges, playing fields, rubbish tips, June to November.
A tall, shaggy, scaly fungus, 8–25 cm (3–10 inches) high. Cap almost
cylindrical at first, white and covered with scales.
Opens to resemble a limp umbrella. Gills white at
first, then pink to black as the cap opens, finally
dissolving into an inky fluid. Stem white and
smooth with a small white ring at first.

The shaggy inkcap has a
preference for grassland that
is managed by
humans rather than
animals. It can often
be found in large
numbers in the
short mown grass by

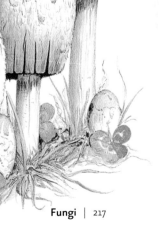

roadsides, even on roundabouts and the central reservations of dual carriageways. It comes up like a white busby and can scarcely be mistaken for any other species, save perhaps its close relative Coprinus atramentarius. This too is edible, but can produce nausea if eaten together with alcohol. Coprinus atramentarius can be distinguished by its dirty grey colour, its absence of scales, its generally more slender build and lack of ring.

The shaggy inkcap should be gathered whilst the cap is still closed and the gills pale, and should be cooked as soon as possible after picking, before the cap starts to dissolve. Remove dirt by wiping with a damp cloth.

Once the stems have been removed, the caps can be fried quickly in oil or butter, or deep-fried in breadcrumbs. Or you can bake them in a very slow casserole with cream or a mustard-flavoured roux for up to one hour. The taste is pleasant and mild, a little like shellfish in texture, but perhaps too innocuous for some palates. Alternatively, a nice conceit is to open a cap so that it resembles a starfish, remove the stem and place it on top of a raw egg in a dish. Then bake in a medium oven for 15 minutes.

Shaggy inkcap ketchup

A good way to capitalise on the deliquescent nature of the shaggy inkcap is to turn them into ketchup. Put the young caps into an earthenware jar, pack them down well and strew each layer with salt. When the jar is full put it in the oven, and simmer for an hour or two, being careful not to lose too much liquid by evaporation. Then strain through muslin, and for each quart of liquid add an ounce of black pepper and a scrape of nutmeg. Boil up again, strain into clean (preferably sterilised) bottles and seal well. The ketchup will keep indefinitely, but should be used quickly once opened.

Red-staining Inocybe

Inocybe patouillardii

☠ POISONOUS

Uncommon in woodland glades, parks, etc.
Cap 5–7 cm (2–3 inches), conical. Gills,
stipe and flesh whitish, but soon reddening
with age or bruising. Smells fruity. Many
inocybe species are toxic, but most grow in
woodland habitats, not in the open
grassland favoured by the fairy-ring
champignon. The most seriously
poisonous member of the family, red-
staining inocybe, is unfortunately sometimes an exception. Avoid all
inocybes.

Galerina mutabilis

Found in clusters on tree stumps from April
onwards. Cap 2–8 cm (1–3 inches) across, dark
brown and slightly sticky when damp, drying from the
centre to a pale chamois-leather colour. Gills
cinnamon. Stem dark brown and scaly up to the
prominent ring; above ring, pale brown and smooth.

One of the earliest fungi to appear, and difficult to confuse
with any other species if it is picked in the spring. Although
the caps are rather small and thin-fleshed, the clusters can
contain literally hundreds, and certainly enough for a good
meal. The fungus has an agreeable flavour, and is excellent
for flavouring soups and stews, to which it gives a rich
brown colour.

Cep
Boletus edulis

Quite common in rides and clearings in all sorts of woods, especially beech, August to November. Cap, brown, dry and smooth, 5–25 cm (2–10 inches) across. Gills in *Boletus* are replaced by pores, much like sponge rubber in appearance, and in *Boletus edulis* they are yellow to olive-brown in colour. Stem short and bulging, pale brown streaked with white. No ring. Flesh white, firm and pleasant-smelling.

All members of the Boletus family are distinguishable by their 'gills', which are a spongy mass of fine tubes beneath the cap. The cep has the additional distinction of looking exactly like a glossy penny bun, to which it is often compared. Alternative names include penny bun, king bolete and porcini.

Ceps are one of the most famous of all edible fungi, and at one time there were six different varieties for sale at Covent Garden. Unfortunately they are equally well liked by insects, so it is as well to cut the caps in half before cooking to check that they are not infested. To prepare for cooking remove the stem, and scoop away the pores with a spoon (unless they are very young and firm).

They are delicious sliced and eaten raw, but there is a prodigious number of recipes for ceps. They can be sliced and fried in oil for a few minutes with a little garlic and parsley. They can be fried with potatoes, or grilled with fish. They are excellent for drying (and indeed in the dried form are quite widely available in delicatessens), and reconstitute well after being soaked in warm water. Dried ceps can also be ground into powder and used as flavouring.

Beetroot and cep soup

This is an attractive old Polish recipe for a soup which is served on Christmas Eve. Make some clear beetroot stock by boiling chopped raw beetroots in water, with bay leaves and peppercorns. Take your sliced ceps and fry in butter with chopped onion and paprika pepper for about five minutes. Take some ravioli-shaped pasta cases and fill with the cep and onion mixture, minced fine. Seal the cases, and bake in the oven until golden-brown. Reheat the beetroot stock, and sharpen to taste with a little vinegar and lemon juice. At the last minute add the hot cases and serve.

Most Boletus species are mild and nutty to taste, and they are amongst the most popular edible fungi in mainland Europe. There are a large number of boletes growing in the British Isles, and all of them have the same foam-like gill structure. A few are indigestible or can cause bad gastric upsets. Luckily all of these are coloured red or purple on pores or stem, and so are easily avoided. None of the edible species described below has this feature.

Bay Bolete
Boletus badius

Quite common in woodland on acid soils, favouring Scots pine. August to November. Similar to Boletus edulis. Cap 7–15 cm (3–6 inches) across, chestnut to chocolate-brown, felt-like when dry but slightly clammy when wet. Pores pale yellow to yellow-green. Stem yellow-brown, stout and often curved and striated. Flesh white to pale yellow, stains pale blue when cut.

Yellow-cracked Bolete

Boletus subtomentosus

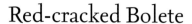

Found in all sorts of wood, especially in moss and on grassy paths, June to October. Cap 5–7 cm (2–3 inches) across, colour variable, olive-yellow to brown; when old the surface is often cracked. Pores bright yellow. Stem yellow-brown, ribbed, tapering towards the base. Flesh soft, yellowish-white, pleasant smelling.

Red-cracked Bolete

Boletus chrysenteron

A common woodland species. Cap colour is variable, usually yellow-brown with a pink layer beneath. Pores yellow to olive, bruising blue. Stem yellow with a reddish tinge. Edible but soggy and can be prone to infestation by maggots.

Devil's Bolete

Boletus satanas

☠ **POISONOUS**

Rare and local, under broadleaved trees in the south of England. Cap large, 8–25 cm (3–10 inches) across, almost hemispherical and entirely white, turning greyish with age. Pores tiny, first yellow then red; bruise blue-green. Stem swollen and covered with red veining. Flesh yellow, very unpleasant smell. Very indigestible, and can cause severe gastric complaints in some people.

Boletus erythropus

Common in woodland clearings on acid soils. Cap large, up to 20 cm (8 inches) across, chestnut to liver-brown in colour. Pores small, round, deep orange-red, blue when bruised. Stem thick and yellow, covered with red spotting. Flesh yellowish, turning intense blue when cut or broken. Little smell or taste. An edible fungus, but probably best avoided because of the possibility of misidentification of B. satanas. Other edible species that can be similarly confused are B. luridus, B. queletii and B. rhodopurpureus.

Gyroporus cyanescens

Rare in woods on poor soil, especially spruce, July to December. Cap 4–10 cm (1¹/₂–4 inches) across, rough, pale ochre in colour. Pores white to pale yellow. Stem stout, velvety, pale ochre. The flesh is white but turns deep blue immediately after cutting.

Slippery Jack
Suillus luteus

Quite common amongst grass in conifer woods, September to November. Cap 6–12 cm (2–5 inches) across, orange-brown, tinged with purple, and slimy to the touch. Pores white to pale yellow. Stem yellow, with a floppy, brownish-purple ring. Flesh yellow, unchanging when cut. Peel before cooking. Will not keep and therefore unsuitable for drying.

Suillus granulatus

Quite common in conifer woods, June to October.
Cap 5–8 cm (2–3 inches) across, slimy, straw-yellow to
leather-brown. Peels easily. Pores yellow to olive, and
when young exudes milky drops. Stem slender, light
yellow, granular, no ring. Flesh yellowish,
unchanging when cut, fruity to smell.
Very susceptible to maggots.

Larch Bolete
Suillus grevillei

Quite common, in larch woods only, June to
November. Cap 4–12 cm (1½–5 inches) across, slimy,
pale yellow. Pores sulphur yellow, bruise brown. Stem
tall, yellowish brown, with a pale ring which soon
disappears. Flesh has the colour and texture of
rhubarb and stains pale lilac on cutting.
Remove skin and tubes before cooking.

Brown Birch Bolete
Leccinum scabrum

Found in grass under birches, July to
November. Cap 5–10 cm (2–4 inches) across,
smooth and greyish-brown, dry, but sticky in
wet weather. Gills white to dirty fawn. Stem
tall, white, flecked with brown or black scales.
Flesh soft, soon becoming moist and
spongy. Usually fairly free of maggots.

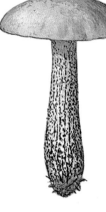

Orange Birch Bolete
Leccinum versipelle

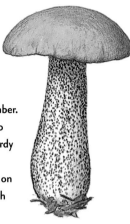

Found under birches and conifers, July to November. Cap 8–18 cm (3–7 inches) across, orange-yellow to yellow-brown. Pores minute, dirty grey. Stem sturdy and tapering towards the cap, slate coloured, scurfy. Flesh white, very slowly turning dirty pink on cutting. Don't be alarmed by the fact that the flesh turns black on cooking.

Russula species

There are over 100 species of *Russula* in Britain. With their brightly coloured caps, they are amongst the most attractive of our native fungi and many (with some exceptions – see below) are good to eat. Often specific to a particular species of tree, *Russulas* are characterised by crumbly flesh.

The *Russulas* are a difficult family, with many species, enormously variable in colouring, and yet too good to omit altogether. Their variability can lead almost any specimen, at some stage in its development, to become one of those vague white-gilled, yellowish, greenish or brownish-capped fungi which are so difficult to tell from the main poisonous species. In fact, none of the *Russulas* themselves are poisonous when cooked – though there are three common species that are poisonous when raw (see p. 228).

Bare-toothed Russula

Bare-toothed Russula

Russula vesca

Russula vesca is probably the easiest of the common species to identify. It grows in all sorts of woods, especially oak and beech, from June to November. The cap is 5–10 cm (2–4 inches) across, and can be coloured anything from pale pink to violet or rusty red. Stem and gills are pure white, and there is no ring or sheath. The best identifying feature is the fact that, when the fungus is mature, one or two millimetres of the margin of the cap are free from skin, and finely grooved with radial veins. Cooked like a *Boletus*, *Russula vesca* is an excellent fungus, firmer than most, and with a mildly nutty taste which has been likened to new potatoes.

Yellow Swamp Russula

Russula claroflava

Common under birch and alder, June to November. Cap 5–12 cm (2–5 inches) across, matt yellow at first, becoming shiny. Gills ochre, stem white, bruising greyish. One of the best of the Russulas, with a fruity smell and a mild taste.

Green-cracking Russula

Russula virescens

Occasional in open broadleaved woodland, especially oak and beech. Cap 4–12 cm (1½–5 inches) across, cream, turning patchy green with age. Gills and flesh creamy-white. This is often regarded as the best edible Russula. Do watch out for maggots.

Russula xerampelina

Found under pines. Cap up to 15 cm (6 inches) across, with no depression, blackish-purple in the centre fading to carmine at edge. Gills ochre, flesh yellowing when cut.

Russula krombholzii

Previously known as R. *atropurpurea*. Common throughout Britain, especially under oak, June to December. Cap 3–10 cm (1–4 inches) across, a striking deep purple in colour with a darker centre. Gills, stem and flesh dull white, smelling slightly of apples.

Charcoal Burner
Russula cyanoxantha

Found under broadleaved trees throughout Britain. Cap 5–15 cm (2–6 inches) across, a mixture of colours ranging from greenish-blue to violet. Gills soft and white. Stem and flesh white, with little or no smell.

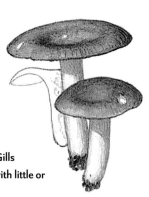

Russula rosea

Found under broadleaved trees, especially beech.
Cap 8–12 cm (3–5 inches) across, slightly depressed in
the centre, a delicate pink fading towards the centre.
Gills and flesh white, with no distinctive smell or taste.

The Sickener

Russula emetica
☠ **POISONOUS**

Common under pine or birch. Cap 5–10 cm
(2–4 inches) across, shiny bright cherry-red or
vermilion. Gills and flesh white, with a fruity smell.
Poisonous when raw and best avoided altogether.

Russula aeruginea

Quite common under birch and conifers. Cap 8–12 cm
(3–5 inches) across, with no central depression, greenish-
grey in colour. Gills forked and yellowish. Stem white, yellowing
slightly with age. Can cause stomach upsets, and best avoided.

Beechwood Sickener

Russula mairei
☠ **POISONOUS**

Similar to the sickener but grows under beeches. Cap 3–7 cm
(1–3 inches) across, matt cherry-red or vermilion. Gills white with a
grey-green tint. Stem white, yellowing at the base. Smells of coconut.

Saffron Milk Cap

Lactarius deliciosus

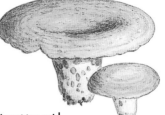

Occurs in pine woods, provided the soil is not too acid, September to November. Funnel-shaped, with a short orange stem and a cap 5–15 cm (2–6 inches) across, orange-red, with darker banding and a depression in the centre. Gills bright orange, crowded. The whole fungus exudes beads of orange milk, which turns green and stains older specimens.

The best of the edible milk caps, as suggested by its Latin name. A popular fungus in parts of Europe, but too rich (and occasionally bitter) for some tastes. The bitterness can be removed by blanching. Once dried, the mushroom can be fried or grilled – the latter is recommended, as it makes the most of the crisp texture. It goes well with fish, and its eye-catching colour make it an attractive addition to any dish.

The saffron milk cap can be confused with two poisonous relatives:

Lactarius helvus

Also found with pine, but distinguished by a lack of bands on the yellow-brown cap, with stem and gills the same colour, and a water-like milk. Smells of fenugreek.

Woolly Milk Cap

Lactarius torminosus

Found with birch, the stem, gills and cap are flesh-pink. The cap does feature darker rings, but the cap has a woolly appearance, and the milk is white.

Giant Puffball

Calvatia gigantea

Meadows, pastures, sometimes under hedges, July to November. A large and roughly spherical fungus, usually 10–30 cm (4–12 inches) across, white, smooth and leathery initially. Flesh solid, spongy, and pure white when young, turning to yellow and dirty green when old. Grows apparently straight from the ground, with little or no stalk.

To come upon one of these suddenly is a memorable experience, only rivalled by the taste of the first mouthful. There is not much point in searching deliberately for them; they are always unexpected, glinting like huge displaced eggs under a hedge or in the corner of a field. It always seems sad to butcher the soft, kid-leather skin, but when you do cut through the flesh, the great flaky slabs of white meat that fall away are just as inviting.

Giant puffballs can grow to a prodigious size. Some have been found over 1 metre (4 ft) in diameter. The usual size is more like a small football, but even this will provide a feast for a large number of people, for every part of the fungus is solid, edible flesh. The important quality to look out for is that this flesh is still pure white. As it ages, puffball flesh turns yellow and then pale brown, becoming progressively less appetising and increasingly indigestible. It finally dissolves into a dust which consists of the reproductive spores. The giant puffball is one of the most fecund of all living organisms, and a single specimen may produce up to seven billion spores. If all of these germinated successfully and produced similar specimens with equally successful spores, their grandchildren would form a mass eight hundred times the volume of the earth.

There is no real need to peel puffballs, though the skin may be too leathery for some tastes. Simply clean them, and slice into 1 cm (½ inch) steaks for frying, grilling or baking. The slices taken from the smoother, more rubbery flesh near the top of the fungus are like sweetbreads; the more crumbly steaks from near the base are softer and less succulent, a little like an omelette or toasted marshmallow.

Even with small specimens you are likely to be left with some perfectly good surplus flesh, and some collectors have experimented with deep-freezing this. The slices can be frozen fresh, but tend to become rather soggy on thawing. Better results are obtained by coating them in egg and breadcrumbs, frying them, and then freezing.

Perhaps the answer is not to pick the whole puffball at once, but to follow the practice recommended by one Victorian writer:

'We have known specimens to grow amongst cabbages in a kitchen garden, and when such is the case it may be left standing, slices being cut off as required until the whole is consumed.'

Stuffed puffball

Hollow out the puffball until there is a shell about 2.5 cm (1 inch) thick remaining. Fill it with a mixture of mince, herbs, rice and the crumbled-up hollowings. Wrap with bacon and metal foil and bake in a medium oven for about one hour. The very heavy aroma during cooking may put some people off, but the ball resembles a roast turkey when it emerges from the oven

Fried puffball steaks

1 medium-sized giant puffball
50 g (2 oz) seasoned flour
1 egg
Water
1 cupful breadcrumbs
8 rashers of bacon (optional)
Butter or vegetable oil (if not using bacon)

1 Wipe the puffball clean, and cut unto slices about 1 cm (½ inch) thick, checking that they are clear of any yellowish tinge.
2 Make a batter by beating the flour and egg together until smooth, then slowly adding water until the mixture is the consistency of single cream.
3 Dip each side of the puffball steaks into the batter, then into the breadcrumbs spread into a shallow dish. Toasting the breadcrumbs beforehand makes a crunchy alternative.
4 Leave the battered, crumbed steaks to one side for a few minutes while you fry the bacon.
5 Remove the bacon from the pan, and fry the puffball slices in the fat (or in vegetable oil or butter).
6 Serve with the bacon, if using.

There are a number of different species of puffball growing in the British Isles, all resembling more or less miniature versions of the giant puffball. All are edible when young and white-fleshed, though they tend to be rubbery in texture and lack the exquisite taste of the giant species. But there is a species of a related family, the common earthball (*Scleroderma citrinum*) which can cause gastric upsets if eaten in quantity. This resembles a puffball in shape, but its surface is hard, brown and scaly. So it is as well to pick only those puffballs which are white or creamy, and relatively smooth-skinned.

It is usual to peel these smaller balls, as the skin can be tougher than the giant puffball's. This, together with the cutting of the base, will tell you if the flesh is white inside. These smaller balls can be cooked like *Calvatia gigantea*, or stewed whole in milk.

The commonest species is the common puffball.

Common Puffball

Lycoperdon perlatum

Pastures, heaths and sometimes woods, June to November. 2–7 cm (1–3 inches) across, more pear-shaped than spherical, skin white to cream when young, usually covered with tiny, spiny pimples.

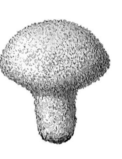

Calvatia utriformis

Lawns, pastures and sand dunes. About 3–7 cm (1–3 inches) across, with no stipe. Entirely white or cream in colour, with a slightly mealy surface.

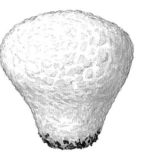

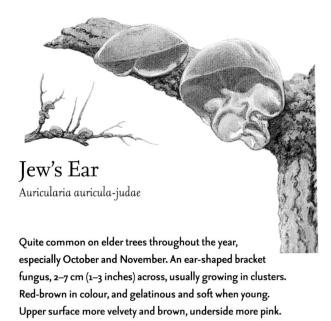

Jew's Ear

Auricularia auricula-judae

**Quite common on elder trees throughout the year,
especially October and November. An ear-shaped bracket
fungus, 2–7 cm (1–3 inches) across, usually growing in clusters.
Red-brown in colour, and gelatinous and soft when young.
Upper surface more velvety and brown, underside more pink.**

I can imagine no food more forbidding in appearance than
the Jew's ear fungus. It hangs in folds from decaying elder
branches like slices off some ageing kidney, clammy and
jelly-like to the touch. It is no fungus to leave around the
house if you have sensitive relatives, or even to forget about
in your own pocket.

But it is a good edible species for all that, and is much
prized in China, where a related species is grown for food on
oak palings. It was also valued by the old herbalists (as *fungus
sambuci*) as a poultice for inflamed eyes, though apparently
not sufficiently to warrant a more complimentary name.
Anti-Semitism in the Middle Ages meant that 'Jew's meat'
was a deprecatory term for all fungi, though the name of this
species may contain an oblique reference to Judas, who
reputedly hanged himself from an elder tree.

Jew's ear should be gathered whilst it is still soft and
moist (it turns rock-hard with age) and cut from the tree

with a knife. Discard all of the tough stalk, wash it well, and slice it finely, for although the translucent flesh is thin it can be tough and indigestible. Stew for a good three-quarters of an hour in stock or milk, and serve with plenty of pepper. The result is crisp and not unlike a seaweed. It can be dried, and is best ground to a powder and used as a flavouring.

Chinese-style Auricularia soup

An unusual sweet soup is made with the very similar cloud ear fungus (Auricularia polytricha) in China, and the recipe is equally suitable for the Jew's ear fungus. Clean and soak 25 g (1 oz) of the fungus and chop roughly. Heat 800 g (2 lb) of brown sugar crystals in 500 ml (1 pint) of water until the sugar melts and the mixture is almost boiling. Drain the ears, add to the syrup and steam for $1^1/_2$ hours. Serve hot or cold.

Lichens

Iceland Moss
Cetraria islandica

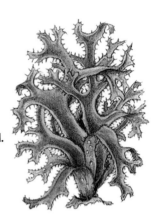

This rust-brown lichen grows amongst the heather and other ground plants on moorlands in Scotland and the north of England.

An edible jelly is sometimes made by boiling the plant, which is first soaked in water to remove the bitter flavour.

Rock Tripe
Umbilicaria pustulata

This is a strange lichen, growing like a mat of pebbles on rocks and walls in western regions of Britain.

It is edible if cooked like a seaweed, and some arctic explorers have survived off it for weeks on end. Yet they have more praise for its powers of nourishment than for its taste; one gives the rather forbidding description, 'a little like tapioca with a slight flavouring of liquorice'.

Seaweeds

Although they reproduce by spores, not flowers and seeds, seaweeds have seasons of growth like other plants. They produce shoots in the spring, grow quickly and luxuriantly during the summer, and wither in the winter. The best months to gather most seaweeds are May and June.

Seaweeds obtain their food entirely from the surrounding sea water and do not have roots in the conventional sense. However, they do have hold-fasts, by which they attach themselves to rocks and stones, and from which the stem-like part, or stipe, grows. The weed itself can regenerate from a cut stipe, provided the cut is not too near the hold-fast. So if you are cutting seaweed rather than gathering leaves which have been washed free of their moorings, leave plenty of stipe so that the weed can grow again.

Some cooking hints

There are a number of basic ways of dealing with all seaweeds:
- Before eating any seaweed always wash thoroughly in fresh water to remove sand, shells and other shoreline debris which may have stuck to it.
- Slice them very thin and serve raw as a salad. A Chinese-style dressing of soy sauce, vinegar and a little sugar is a good accompaniment.
- Slice them a little less thinly, and stir-fry in sesame or sunflower oil for about 5 minutes, or in more oil at a higher temperature, until they are crisp on the outside.

- Add larger pieces to soups and stews to thicken them. Most seaweeds contain alginates, a kind of vegetable gelatine, which are released during prolonged cooking.

Seaweeds are low in calories but rich in minerals, particularly iodides, and you may take a little while to get used to their flavours. But do give them a fair chance: they are intriguing foods and undeserving of their somewhat freakish reputation.

Sea Lettuce
Ulva lactuca

Quite common on all types of shore, at all tidal levels, especially in places where water runs into the sea. Broad, tough, crumpled green fronds, 10–30 cm (4–12 inches) across, attached to stones and rocks.

One of the more pleasant seaweeds served raw, especially chopped, and served Japanese-style with soy sauce and rice vinegar.

Dabberlocks
Alaria esculenta

Commonest on exposed shores of Atlantic and North Sea coasts, where it takes the place of *Laminaria digitata* (below). Short stem, narrow, slightly wavy blade 0.5–3 m (1½–10 ft) long. Fronds may appear feathery. Yellowish-olive to reddish-brown.

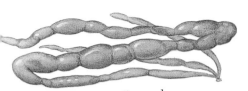

Gutweed

Gutweed

Dabberlocks

Enteromorpha intestinalis

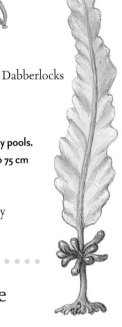

Abundant on salt marshes and in dikes and rocky pools.
Inflated green tube, irregularly constricted, up to 75 cm
(30 inches) long.

A weed which should be picked in the early
spring, and stir-fried until crisp.

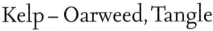

Kelp – Oarweed, Tangle

Laminaria digitata

Grows at and just below the low-water mark on rocky shores all
round the coast, often forming extensive 'meadows' at low water.
Also found attached to small stones on muddy and sandy flats. Blade
up to 2 m (6 ft) long, splits into fingers as it matures.

The young stipes of this weed used
to be sold in Scotland under the
name of 'tangle'. One writer
describes their taste as resembling
that of peanuts. A composite jelly,
made from this weed and dulse and
called *pain des algues*, used to be prepared
in the west of France.

Kelp – Sea Belt, Poor-man's Weather-glass
Laminaria saccharina

Another common kelp, found at the low-water mark on rocky shores all around the coast. A short slender stem and a ribbon-like blade, up to 4 m (13 ft) long, with crinkled edges.

As well as a salad vegetable, this kelp is used as a source of alginates.

Bladder Wrack, Popweed
Fucus vesiculosus

Abundant on the middle shore, into estuaries, and unmistakable for its inflated bladders. Frond up to 1 m (3 ft) long, characterised by prominent midrib and gas bladders. Dark olive-brown.

This common seaweed can be washed, simmered in a little water and served as a green vegetable.

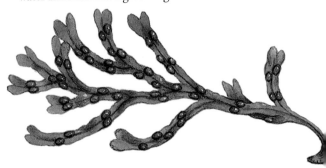

Dulse

Palmaria palmata

Abundant on stones on the middle and lower shores, on the North Sea and northern Atlantic coasts. A tough, flat frond 10–30 cm (4–12 inches) long. Dark red, but can look purple under water.

Dulse has been eaten raw as a salad, and in New England the dried fronds are used as a relish. It is also occasionally grazed by sheep and cattle. It is very tough, and as a cooked vegetable needs up to five hours' simmering.

• •

Pepper Dulse

Laurencia pinnatifida

An infrequent weed which forms dense tufts in rock crevices on the middle shore. Flattened fronds, 7–20 cm (3–8 inches), with alternate branches dividing into smaller branchlets. Brownish-purple.

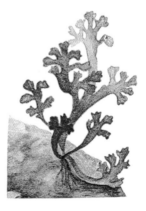

Pepper dulse is very pungent and is usually used as a condiment. In Iceland it has been employed as a substitute for chewing tobacco.

Purple Laver

Porphyra umbilicalis

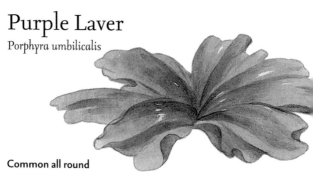

**Common all round
Britain, especially on exposed shores on the west coast. Grows on
rock and stones at most levels of the beach, especially where the
stones are likely to be covered with sand. The fronds are thin,
irregularly shaped membranes, 20 cm (8 inches) across, greenish
when young, becoming purplish-red.**

In the southwest of Wales laver is considered a great
delicacy, and it sells briskly in many food shops to those who
don't want the bother of gathering it for themselves.

Yet it is one of the easier seaweeds to find and recognise,
its translucent purple fronds liable to crop up on almost all
levels of the shore. In Asia *Porphyra* species are cultivated,
and they are best known by the Japanese name nori. Bundles
of bamboo are placed on the sea bottom, just offshore, and
transferred to fresh river water once the weed has
established itself. In these conditions the plant apparently
grows softer and more extensive fronds. In Japan, China and
Korea, nori is widely used, in soups and stews, as a covering
round rice balls, and in pickles and preserves.

In Britain there have been two classic traditional uses:
laverbread, and laver sauce for mutton.

Laverbread

The first stage in any laver recipe is to reduce the
weed to a sort of rough purée. First wash it well and
then simmer in a little water until it is like well-

cooked spinach. This is best done in a double saucepan as the laver sticks easily. This mush, if transferred to a jar, will keep well for several days. It is this puree which is sold in Wales under the name of laverbread. It ends up in the place you would least expect it – on the breakfast table, rolled in oatmeal and fried in bacon fat.

Laver sauce

Beat up two cupfuls of the laver purée with 25 g (1 oz) of butter and the juice of one Seville orange.

Carrageen, Irish Moss

Chondrus crispus

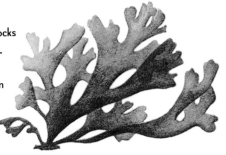

Widespread on stones and rocks on temperate Atlantic shores. Grows in clusters of purple-brown fronds, usually 5–15 cm (2–6 inches) in length. These have a distinctly flat stalk, and branch repeatedly into a rough fan shape.

Carrageen is an important source of alginates – vegetable gelatines – which are used for thickening soups, emulsifying ice-creams and setting jellies. They can also be made into thin durable films for use as edible sausage skins.

You can find carrageen on almost any western or southern shore. It is best gathered young, in April or May, and either used immediately or carefully dried. To use the weed fresh, wash it well, add one cup of weed to three cups of milk or water, and add sugar and flavouring to taste. Then simmer slowly until most of the weed has dissolved. Remove any undissolved fragments and pour into a mould to set. This produces a basic caragean blancmange or jelly, depending on whether you use milk or water. Ginger is good as a flavouring, and can be added in the form of the chopped root, or as ground powder, during the simmering of the weed.

To dry the weed, wash it well, and then lay it out to dry on a wind-free surface out of doors. Wash it from time to time with fresh water, or simply leave it in the rain. After a while it will become bleached to a creamy-white colour. Trim off any tough stalks, dry thoroughly indoors, and then store in bags. The dried weed can be used exactly as if it were fresh.

Gigartina stellata

Common and often abundant on the middle and lower shore, especially on the west coast.

Can be used to make a jelly base.

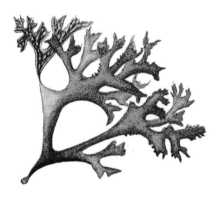

SHELLFISH

It is believed that many of the more bloodcurdling superstitions associated with the mandrake – in particular its power to flee from prospective pickers on leg-like roots, or kill them off with its notorious shriek – were invented by professional Greek herb pickers, who were anxious to keep amateurs away from their livelihood. The same is probably true of many of the stories concerning the poisonousness of shellfish out of season. Shellfish are one of the lifelines by which coastal dwellers hang on to a measure of independence round the year. Yet they are also one of the most tempting of wild foods that are there just for the picking. Unhappily for the professionals, the next generation of pickings is being spawned just when the holidaymakers are trooping out to the mudflats with their buckets and spades. No wonder, then, that the gentle warnings of superstition, the one sort of 'keep out' notice permissible on public land, are propped up rather more than they would be by facts alone.

In fact every sort of fish is slightly out of condition during the breeding season, but none need be poisonous, not even shellfish. This is not to say that there are no good reasons for leaving shellfish alone during the summer months. Molluscs are highly susceptible to disease and temperature change, and unless the largest possible numbers are allowed to spawn freely, their survival rate will be low.

And ironically, the way we are currently treating our coastal waters may yet turn the story into sound advice. Bivalve molluscs (with shells in two hinged halves like castanets) feed by pumping water through their shells and filtering out the food particles. In doing this they may also filter out sewage particles and the enteric bacteria which are associated with them. During the warm weather which corresponds to the off-season these bacteria can multiply alarmingly, up to a level which can cause food poisoning in humans. Unfortunately this is particularly true of large bivalves like mussels and oysters, which filter a great deal of water each day, and sometimes seem to relish the warm, soupy conditions near sewage outlets.

So shellfish should be approached with caution, but not with trepidation, and with the knowledge that it is not some sinister springtime sap that makes them chancy during the warm months, but our own disgusting habits.

Rules

If you keep to these few rules, you will never need a stomach pump.

1 Never gather shellfish close to human dwellings, or anywhere where sewage or refuse is pumped into the sea.

2 Always wash them well, outside and in, in clean water.

3 Check that all your specimens are alive immediately before cooking them. Shellfish decompose very quickly after death, and a dead mollusc is more dangerous than a dirty one. To tell if a bivalve shellfish is alive, gently force its shell open a fraction of an inch. It should shut again quickly as soon as you take off the pressure. If it is already open, opens wide with ease, or fails to shut again, it is safer to assume that it is dead.

Common Limpet

Patella vulgata

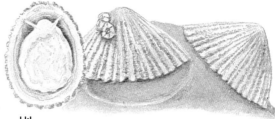

Common on rocky shores round all British coasts. Limpets are shaped like flat cones and cling to rocks. Shell up to 6 cm (2¹/₂ inches) across.

Limpets graze on algae when the tide is in, returning to their individual resting places as the tide recedes. The common limpet can grow quite large, but it is normally somewhat smaller, and consequently a fair number – and a fair degree of scrambling – are needed to gather enough for a meal. Do not pick them from piers or jetties, but from out-of-town rocks that are covered daily by the tide. They can be prised from the rocks with a knife.

Soak them and then boil them, like cockles, until the meat floats free of the shell. Be warned, though: limpets can be very tough, and they may need considerable further simmering or baking. In the Isle of Man limpets used to be fried at Easter.

Common Periwinkle, Winkle

Littorina littorea

Widely distributed round all British coasts. Common on rocks and weeds on the middle shore. A sharply pointed shell, 1–2.5 cm (¹/₂–1 inch) high, spiralled like a tiny whelk, and normally dark grey in colour.

You will not need to spend very long unravelling a bowl of winkles from their tortuous shells before you appreciate why the process produced a new verb of extrication for the English language.

Judged purely as food, winkles do not have much to commend them. They have none of the rich flavour of mussels or the muscular texture of whelks. You need a dozen to provide a single mouthful. The joy of winkle eating lies wholly in the challenge of getting the things out of their shells, and, for the experienced, in the leisurely ritual of the pin and the twist. In Food in England, Dorothy Hartley describes a delightful encounter with a connoisseur:

> 'I learnt "winkles" from a night watchman. He used to sit by his big red coke fire-bucket, a bit of folded blanket over his knees, his mug of hot tea, and a little enamel bowl full of winkles. And he would turn up the little tab-end at the bottom of his waistcoat, pull out a long pin, and take a winkle ... And then he would chuck the empty shell neatly over his shoulder into the canal with a tiny "plop". He did it quite slowly, and he always paused (I can see him now, red in the fire-light, head aslant, his huge hand still half-open, curved like a hoary brown shell). He always paused just that second till he heard the tiny plop, before he bent and picked up the next winkle. His old woman had put him "a reet proper breakfast", and he had a basket with a bottle in it. But, as he said, "Winkles, they do pass the time along very pleasantly." '

You can find winkles on almost every stretch of rocky or weedy shore between high and low tide-marks. They are often in quite large colonies, and can be easily gathered. To clean the sand and grit out from them thoroughly, soak them in fresh water for about twelve hours. Then cook them by plunging them into boiling water and simmering for about ten minutes.

Then eat them like the night watchman, leisurely, with a long pin, and perhaps a little salt and vinegar at the side. The whole fish is edible, except for the tiny mica-like plate at the mouth of the shell, which should be removed with your pin before you winkle out the flesh.

- -

Common Mussel, Blue Mussel
Mytilus edulis

Found on all coasts on rocks from the middle shore down. The edible mussel is up to 10 cm (4 inches) long and has a blue-black shell with a pearly, whitish lining.

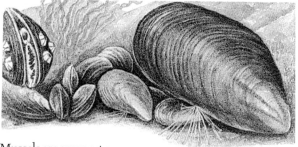

Mussels are amongst our commonest and most delectable shellfish. But they are also responsible for most cases of shellfish poisoning. If you follow the rules given on p. 246 you are unlikely to eat a bad mussel. Gather them from clean stony shores at low tide outside the summer months, let them stand through at least two changes of fresh tap-water, and check that each one is still alive before cooking.

If you only have a few, try baking them in their shells in hot ash, and popping in a mixture of butter garlic and parsley as the shells open.

- -

Scallop
Pecten maximus

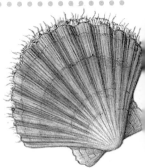

The scallop has a reddish-brown shell with characteristic ribs, and may measure up to 15 cm (6 inches) across.

This is the classic shell that came to be the oil company's symbol. You find them occasionally on the lower shore, on that strip of sand that is only uncovered during very low tides.

Like clams, scallops need careful cooking. After washing and scalding, cut away the white and orange flesh, dust with flour or breadcrumbs and fry for about five minutes. They have a superbly fleshy, almost poultry-like flavour.

- -

Oyster
Ostrea edulis

The oyster shell is smooth and white to begin with, but as it ages it becomes grey and scaly. It, too, may measure as much as 15 cm (6 inches) across.

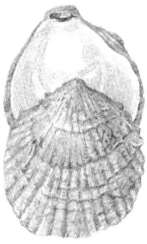

Oysters have not always been the expensive delicacy that they are now. For centuries they were one of the great staples of working-class diet. In the latter half of the nineteenth century prices suddenly rocketed, and there is little doubt that the cause was the irresponsible over-harvesting of the beds to meet the demands of expanding townships.

Today you will be lucky to find many wild oysters. The ones that still remain round our coasts are mostly under cultivation in private beds. So if you should chance upon one, clinging to a rock in some estuary or creek, best leave it where it is. But if eat it you must, there is only one way: raw, with lemon and tabasco sauce.

• •

Cockle
Cerastoderma edule

Widely distributed round all coasts. Common in sand or sandy mud on the middle shore. A rather dumpy, globular shell up to 6 cm (2¹/₂ inches) across. The two halves are heavily ribbed and are pale brown to grey-blue in colour.

Just after the tide has gone out over the vast salt marshes on the north Norfolk coast, you will sometimes see a cluster of enormous slate-coloured cockles strewn across the muddy sand like dice. These are the famous 'Stiffkey blues', the best and fattest cockles of all.

To find any cockles, big or small, as conspicuously displayed as this is a rare piece of luck. More often they are 2–8 centimetres under the surface. There is no simple rule about where they can be found between the tidelines. A vein of mud in the sand is a good sign; so is a green film of plankton over the surface. But the only sure test is to scratch about and see if they are there. Hands will do if you only want a few, but a rake with blunted points is the best way of pulling them out of the sand quickly. Gather them into a bucket or bag. Do not throw them: the shells break easily, and a broken cockle is very quickly a dead one. Don't pick any specimen less than 2 cm across either. It's scarcely worth the bother. And cockles, like all shellfish, wage a constant battle for survival against pollution and over-picking. If the young are taken before they have had a chance to spawn then the battle is bound to be a losing one. Many stretches of coast have experienced shellfish droughts recently, and though there is probably no single explanation, the over-picking of immature shells is certainly a contributing factor.

When you have all the cockles you want, take them home and wash off the superficial mud and sand. Let them rinse themselves through in a bucket of clean, fresh water for at least six hours, and preferably overnight. Then drop them into a saucepan of boiling water, checking each one for signs of life immediately before. They will quickly open, and be thoroughly cooked within five minutes.

The results can be made into soups or pies, or eaten plain as soon as they have been strained from the water. Try experimenting with sauces to go with the freshly cooked fish. A friend of mine once concocted one out of the improbable ingredients of yoghurt, mustard and horse-radish, and it made a wonderfully tart, silky foil to the springy flesh of the cockles. One eighteenth-century cookery book recommends that the cooked fish should be stuffed into slits in marsh lamb, as if the meat were larded with them.

Cockles and bacon

Cook the bacon very crisp first, then remove it from the pan and fry the cockles in its fat. Serve them together on toast with plenty of pepper.

• •

Clam, Sand Gaper

Mya arenaria

Widely distributed. Common in sand and sandy mud on the middle and lower shore. An oval shell not unlike a large mussel in shape, up to 12.5 cm (5 inches) across, coloured grey or brownish.

These large mussel-like shells have protruding trunks, which are siphons through which the shellfish feed whilst they are buried. The siphons can be extended up to 30 cm (1 foot) in length.

Gather them into a bucket, but do not pick any small specimens. Clams are big enough to need substantially more cooking than most shellfish. As with cockles, let them rinse themselves through in a bucket of clean, fresh water for at least six hours, and preferably overnight. Then scald them in boiling water for about ten minutes and remove them from their shells. The siphon is usually trimmed off, and the remaining meat fried or baked for a further half an hour, or simply boiled until tender and served with a sauce.

Clam chowder

Simmer together chopped clams, fried pieces of pork, onion and potato, with milk added as the soup comes off the boil.

GLOSSARY

Alternate leaves – one leaf per node, successive ones on opposite sides of the stem

Annual – any plant that germinates from seed, grows to maturity and produces new seed all within one year or growing season

Basal leaves – leaves growing a the bottom of the stem

Biennial – a plant which takes more than one but less than two years to complete its life cycle, not flowering in the first year

Boss – protuberance or swelling, often at base of trunk

Bracts – modified leaves growing close to a flower or flowerhead and protecting it

Bulb – swollen underground food-storage organ for the dormant plant, consisting of condensed stem and succulent scale-like leaves

Calyx – ring of petal-like sepals (usually green) which protect the flower when in bud

Catkin – drooping spike bearing much-reduced flowers, generally wind-pollinated, e.g. hazel

Compound leaves – leaves made up of separate leaflets

Drupelet – one part of a compound fruit (e.g. blackberry, raspberry), consisting of a small fleshy fruit containing a seed enclosed in a hard coat

Fissured bark – deeply cracked bark

Floret – group of tiny flowers

Flower-head – group of tightly packed flowers

Leaflet – a division of a compound leaf

Linear leaves – long and narrow leaves

Lobed leaves – leaves with rounded projections

Mast – fruit of forest trees such as beech, oak, etc

Naturalised – an alien plant which has established a self-sustaining population

Nodes – thickened parts of the stem which may grow opposite each other, or be alternate up the stem

Odd-pinnate – pinnate leaf with a single terminal leaflet

Perennial – a plant that lives from year to year, generally with woody stems or organs (tubers, corms, bulbs)

Pinnate leaves – leaves with leaflets growing along either side of central vein

Reflexed – bent down or back

Rhizomes – underground stems

Rosette – leaves spreading from the centre

Runners – stems which grow horizontally above or below the ground and develop small roots and new plants at their tips

Sepal – any of the separate parts of the calyx

Shrub – a woody plant that is not a tree

Simple leaves – leaves with undivided blades, not compound leaves

Spike – flowerhead in which all the flowers are attached to a single column, with no individual flower stalks

Stamen – male part of flower, consisting of a tall, thin stalk or filament with an enlarged part (the anther) at the top containing pollen

Stigma – female, often feathery, part of style where pollen lands from a male flower during pollination

Stipe – stalk bearing reproductive structure in plants, especially the stalk bearing the cap of a mushroom

Style – tall column at the centre of a flower, bearing the stigma

Succulent – a plant with thick, fleshy leaves or stems

Toothed leaves – jagged-edged leaves

Tree – a woody plant, usually more than 5 m (16 ft) high, with a single trunk

Trefoil – plants having leaves divided into three leaflets

Tuber – swollen roots or underground stems

Umbel – many flowers arising from the same point on a stalk to form a flat-topped umbrella shape, e.g. cow parsley

Whorls – several leaves growing round the stem at each node

SOURCES, REFERENCES AND FURTHER READING

General and historical

Austin, Thomas (ed.), Two Fifteenth Century Cook Books. Early English Text Society, 1888.

Bottero, Jean, The Oldest Cuisine in the World: Cooking in Mesopotamia. University of Chicago Press, 2004.

Brothwell, Don and Patricia, Food in Antiquity. Expanded edition, Johns Hopkins University Press, 1998.

Culpeper, Nicholas, The Complete Herbal, 1653.

Drummond, C. and Wilbraham, Anne, The Englishman's Food. Jonathan Cape, 1957.

Evelyn, John, Acetaria: a Discourse of Sallets, 1699. Facsimile, 1982

Fine, Gary Allen, Morel Tales: The Culture of Mushrooming. Harvard University Press, 1998.

Forsyth, A. A., British Poisonous Plants. Revised edition, Ministry of Agriculture, Fisheries & Food, 1986.

Gerard, John, The Herbal. Revised and enlarged by Thomas Johnson, 1633. Facsimile edition, Dover, New York, 1975.

Giles, W. F., Our vegetables, whence they came. Royal Horticultural Society Journal, vol. 69, 1944.

Godwin, H., The History of the British Flora. 2nd edition, Cambridge University Press, 1975.

Greenoak, Francesca, Forgotten Fruit. Deutsch, 1983.

Grigson, Geoffrey, The Englishman's Flora, 1955. Revised edition, Helicon, 1996.

Grigson, Geoffrey, A Herbal of All Sorts. Phoenix House, 1959.

Grigson, Jane, Jane Grigson's Fruit Book. Joseph, 1982.

Grigson, Jane, Jane Grigson's Vegetable Book. Joseph, 1978.

Hartley, Dorothy, Food in England. Macdonald, 1954.

Helbaek, H., Studying the diet of ancient man. Archaeology vol. 14, 1961.

Henslow, G., The origin and history of our garden vegetables. Royal Horticultural Society Journal, vols. 36, 37, 1910–11.

Hutchins, Sheila, English Recipes. Methuen, 1967.

Hyams, Edward, Plants in the Service of Man. Dent, 1971.

Johnson, Charles, The Useful Plants of Great Britain, 1862.

Juniper, Barrie, and Mabberley, David, The Story of the Apple. Timber Press, 2006.

Lovelock, Yann, The Vegetable Book: an Unnatural History. Allen & Unwin, 1972.

Markham, Gervase, The English Hus-Wife, 1615.

Mabey, Richard, Flora Britannica. Sinclair-Stevenson, 1996.

Mead, W. E., The English Medieval Feast. Allen & Unwin, 1931.

North, Pamela, Poisonous Plants and Fungi. Blandford Press, 1967.

Pirie, N. W., Food Resources: Conventional and Novel. 2nd edition, Penguin, 1976.

Prendergast, Hew and Sanderson, Helen, Britain's Wild Harvest. Royal Botanic Gardens, 2004.

Salisbury, Sir Edward, Weeds and Aliens. 2nd edition, Collins, 1964.

Shulman, Alix Kates, Drinking the Rain. Farrar Straus & Giroux, 1995.

Sole, William, Menthae Britannicae, 1798.

Stearn, W. T., The origin and later development of cultivated plants. Royal Horticultural Society Journal, vol. 90, 1965.

Stevenson, Violet (ed.), A Modern Herbal. Octopus Books, 1974.

Thoreau, Henry David, *Wild Fruits: Thoreau's Rediscovered Last Manuscript*. W. W. Norton, 1999.

Tudge, Colin, *Future Cook*. Beasley, 1980.

Turner, William, *The Herbal*, 1568.

Vaughan, J. G. and Geissler, C., *The New Oxford Book of Food Plants*. Oxford University Press, 1997.

Wallis, T. E., *Textbook of Pharmacognosy*. 5th edition, Churchill, 1967.

White, Florence, *Good Things in England*. Jonathan Cape, 1962.

Wilson, C. Anne, *Food and Drink in Britain*. Constable, 1973.

Wild food guides
British and European

Burrows, Ian, *Food from the Wild*. New Holland, 2005.

Carluccio, Antonio, *The Complete Mushroom Book: the Quiet Hunt*. Quadrille Publishing, 2003.

Eley, Geoffrey, *Wild Fruits and Nuts*. EP Publishing, 1976.

Eley, Geoffrey, *101 Wild Plants for the Kitchen*. EP Publishing, 1977.

Ellis, Lesley, *Simply Seaweed*. Grub Street, 1998.

Fearnley-Whittingstall, Hugh, *A Cook on the Wild Side*. Boxtree, 1997.

Fern, Ken, *Plants for a Future: Edible and Useful Plants for a Healthier World*. Permanent Publications, 1997.

Hatfield, Audrey Wynne, *How to Enjoy Your Weeds*, 1969. New edition, Plum Tree, 1999.

Hill, Jason, *The Wild Foods of Britain*. 3rd edition, A. & C. Black, 1944.

Jordan, Michael, *A Guide to Wild Plants*. Millington, 1976.

Loewenfeld, Claire, and Back, Philippa, *The Complete Book of Herbs and Spices*. 2nd edition, David & Charles, 1974.

Mauduit, Vicomte de, *They Can't Ration These*.
Michael Joseph, 1940. Reprinted, Persephone Books,
2004.
Michael, Pamela, *All Good Things Around Us*. Benn, 1980.
Ministry of Food, *Hedgerow Harvest*, 1943.
Peterson, Vicki, *The Natural Food Catalogue*.
Macdonald & Jane's, 1978.
Phillips, Roger, *Wild Food*. Pan Books, 1983.
Richardson, Rosamond, *Hedgerow Cookery*. Penguin, 1980.
Urquhart, Judy, *Living Off Nature*. Allen Lane, 1980.
White, Florence, *Flowers as Food*. Jonathan Cape, 1939.

Wild food guides
North American

(May be worth consulting, as there is a considerable overlap
between species)

Brackett, B. and Lash, M., *The Wild Gourmet*. David Godine,
1975.
Duke, James A., *Handbook of Edible Weeds*. CRC Press, 2000.
Freitus, Joe, and Haberman, Salli, *Wild Jams and Jellies*.
Stackpole Books, 2005.
Gibbons, Euell, *Stalking the Blue-eyed Scallop*. David McKay,
1966.
Gibbons, Euell, *Stalking the Healthful Herbs*. David McKay,
1966.
Gibbons, Euell, *Stalking the Wild Asparagus*. David McKay,
1962.
Harris, Ben Charles, *Eat the Weeds*. Barre, 1972.
Hitchcock, Susan Tyler, and McIntosh, G. B.,
Gather Ye Wild Things. Harper and Row, 1980.

Lyle, Katie Letcher, The Complete Guide to Edible Wild Plants,
    Mushrooms, Fruits, and Nuts. Lyons Press, 2004.
Peterson, Lee Allen, A Field Guide to Edible Wild Plants.
    Houghton Mifflin, 2000.
Medsger, Oliver Perry, Edible Wild Plants: The Classic Guide to
    the Flavor and Lore of the North American Outdoors.
    Macmillan, 1966. Reprinted, Tab Books, 2001.
Weiner, Michael A., Earth Medicine – Earth Food. Fawcett
    Books, 1991.

Identification guides

Akeroyd, John, Collins Wild Guide: Flowers. Collins, 2004.
Fitter, Alistair, Collins Gem: Trees. Collins, 2004.
Garnweidner, Edmund, Mushrooms and Toadstools.
    Collins, 1994.
Harding, Patrick, Collins Gem: Mushrooms. Collins, 2004.
Harding, Patrick, How to Identify Edible Mushrooms.
    Collins, 1996.
Harding, Patrick, Need to Know? Mushroom Hunting.
    Collins, 2006.
Hayward, Peter. Sea Shore of Britain and Europe. Collins, 2001.
Johnson, Owen, and More, David, Collins Tree Guide.
    Collins, 2004.
Press, Bob, Collins Wild Guide: Trees. Collins, 2005.
Preston-Mafham, Rod, Collins Gem: Seashore. Collins, 2004.
Spooner, Brian, Collins Wild Guide: Mushrooms and Toadstools.
    Collins, 2005.
Sterry, Paul, Complete British Wild Flowers. Collins, 2006.
Walters, Martin, Collins Gem: Wild Flowers. Collins, 2004.

Illustration credits

The publishers wish to acknowledge the following artists:

Marjorie Blamey: pp3, 32–45, 48–57, 60 (bottom), 61–68, 70, 75–79, 84–87, 90– 92, 94 (bottom), 98–106, 109–117, 119, 121, 123, 124, 126–129, 132, 134, 135, 139 (top), 142 (top), 144, 146, 148 (top), 149 (left), 150, 151 (top), 152–158 (top left & bottom), 160–165, 167, 168 (left & right), 169, 174, 175 (top), 177, 178, 180.

Jill Coombs: pp143, 151, 158 (top middle & right), 172, 173 (top).

Victoria Goaman: p171.

Sheila Hadley: pp125 (top), 131, 133, 136–138, 139 (bottom), 142 (bottom), 145 (top).

Marilyn Leader: pp82, 83, 118.

David More: p46.

Valerie Price: pp88, 94 (top), 96, 108, 125 (bottom), 145 (bottom), 148 (bottom), 149 (right), 166, 168 (bottom), 173 (bottom), 175, 179.

Susannah Ray: pp69, 71, 73, 81, 241 (bottom), 243–249, 251–253.

Fiona Silver: p159.

Sue Wickison: pp122, 176.

John Wilkinson: pp60 (top), 93, 187–241 (top), 242, 250.

INDEX

Page numbers in **bold** refer to illustrations